THE MACROPHAGE

A Review of Ultrastructure and Function

THE MACROPHAGE

A Review of Ultrastructure and Function

IAN CARR

*Department of Pathology,
University of Sheffield and Weston Park Hospital,
Sheffield, England*

1973

ACADEMIC PRESS · LONDON · NEW YORK
A Subsidiary of Harcourt Brace Jovanovich, Publishers

ACADEMIC PRESS INC. (LONDON) LTD.
24–28 Oval Road,
London NW1

U.S. Edition published by
ACADEMIC PRESS INC.
111 Fifth Avenue
New York, New York 10003

Library of Congress Catalog Card Number: LCCCN 72–12265
ISBN: 0–12–160550–7

PRINTED IN GREAT BRITAIN BY
W. S. COWELL LTD.
IPSWICH, SUFFOLK

Preface

This book reviews the ultrastructure of the mammalian macrophage, and attempts to correlate ultrastructure with function, laying emphasis where possible on cellular behaviour, rather than on immunological and pathological processes. The literature reviewed related wherever possible to ultrastructure; other areas are less fully covered. The book is intended for senior undergraduate and postgraduate students in biology, and for trainees in pathology and laboratory medicine.

I am grateful to many colleagues, scientific and technical, for help and criticism, especially to Mr P. Norris and Mrs J. Ashmore for technical and photographic help, and to Professors R. Barer and W. A. J. Crane of the University of Sheffield, for their unfailing support of my research, which has been financially aided by the Medical Research Council, and the Cancer Research Campaign (Yorkshire Branch).

Figures 1, 4, 6, 7, 8, 9, 10, 14 and 52 are reproduced from my own published work by permission of the publishers of *Zeitschrift fur Zellforschung und Mikroskopische Anatomie* (Springer Verlag) and Fig. 53 by permission of the publishers of the *Journal of Anatomy* (Cambridge University Press).

Department of Pathology,
University of Sheffield
and Weston Park Hospital,
Sheffield, England   IAN CARR

Contents

Chapter One

INTRODUCTION: THE FREE MACROPHAGES

Introduction

The Russian zoologist Metchnikoff was the first to recognize the importance of a group of cells throughout the metazoan organism, largely responsible for the defence of the organism against attack from without.
There were earlier references to the cells which later came to be called
macrophages; for instance in 1863, von Recklinghausen described cells in
the inflamed cornea and the omentum which were different from pus cells,
and in 1876 von Kupffer described the phagocytes of the liver. Ponfick
(1869) injected cinnabar into the blood stream and showed that it was
taken up by cells in the vicinity of hepatic blood vessels. Cells in the same
area were shown by von Kupffer (1876) to have a stellate appearance after
impregnation with gold chloride and by Wyssokowitch (1887) to phagocytose injected bacteria. A fuller description of the phagocytic properties
and structure of these cells was given by von Kupffer in 1898.

It was however Metchnikoff who really established the importance of
these cells; he studied the uptake of foreign materials in a wide variety of
animals, from starfish to mammals, and emphasized the functional identity
of the cells which took up foreign materials. These he called "macrophages" to distinguish them from the smaller circulating leucocytes or
microphages now widely known as polymorphs. His work is still worth
reading and is readily accessible (reprinted 1968).

The phagocytic functions of the macrophage were extensively studied
by the injection of acid vital dyes which are ingested in large quantities by
macrophages all over the body. The work of Kiyono (1914) and Aschoff
(1924) and others led to the view that the cells which took up these dyes
could be regarded as a system, the reticuloendothelial system of Aschoff.

I

A classic account of the phenomenon of vital staining is that of Cappell (1929–1930). The early history of the macrophage concept is reviewed by Maximow (1928) and by Jaffe (1938). It has recently been suggested that the term reticuloendothelial system refers to a most heterogeneous collection of cells, and that it is better to refer to the macrophages as a group as the mononuclear phagocyte system (van Furth, 1970).

Macrophages are readily isolated alive from the living animal; this led to their being an early and obvious subject to culture. It became clear, notably from the work of Carrel and Ebeling (1922, 1926) that large macrophages could develop in culture from smaller precursors in blood or lymphoreticular organs and that this differentiation was reversible. This type of differentiation has been presumed to occur *in vivo* on the basis of sequences of appearances in fixed preparations. Phase-contrast studies on rabbits' ear preparations carried out by Ebert and Florey (1939) offered further evidence that such transformation could occur in the living animal.

Related to the existence of such transformations was the idea that the phagocytic function of macrophages might somehow vary depending on the stimuli presented by the environment. Lurie (1939) showed that the mature macrophages in tuberculous lesions, phagocytosed carbon more readily than normal macrophages. This hyperfunction was in keeping with the observation of Grogg and Pearse (1952) that tuberculous macrophages had a high content of the enzyme acid phosphatase. Moreover in species with a high resistance to tuberculosis the acid phosphatase content of the macrophages was relatively high.

Recent major advances in knowledge of the macrophage have come from the electron microscope and the use of radioactive isotopes. Application of the former has led to much detailed information on cellular structure. The use of labelled amino acids has led to an understanding of protein synthesis by macrophages, and of thymidine labelling to increased understanding of the lineages of both fixed and free cells.

In the meantime significance was added to the study of the isolated cell by the discovery that a quantitative measure of the phagocytic function of the macrophages of the body, or at least of a large group of them could be obtained by giving an animal an intravenous dose of a colloid, usually carbon and then measuring the blood level of the colloid over a period of time (Biozzi *et al.*, 1953). Moreover, the study of the distribution of administered antigen had led to the belief that the macrophage is of considerable importance in processing antigen. In addition it has been known for a long time that macrophages play an important role in the metabolism of iron and lipid, and are the essential cellular element in many chronic inflammatory lesions.

Terminology

Many other terms have been used to describe the macrophage. Some are of purely historical interest. "Clasmatocyte" (Ranvier, 1890) refers to the fact that some macrophages when observed in culture break off little pieces of their cytoplasm. "Rhagiocrine cell" (Renaut, 1907) refers to the red inclusions which appear within macrophages incubated in neutral red and which were thought to be secretory. Marchand (1924) believed that most macrophages arose from perivascular cells and therefore called them "adventitial cells". The amoeboid macrophages of loose connective tissue were called by Kiyono (1914) "histiocytes"; the term should be restricted to connective tissue macrophages.

The term "reticular cell" has been attached to at least four types of cell—the fibroblasts of lymphoreticular tissues, phagocytic cells lining sinusoids which are best described as macrophages, primitive undifferentiated cells for which the term stem cell seems better, and dendritic reticular cells or dendritic macrophages (Milanesi, 1965a, b; Maruyama and Masuda, 1965). These are the only cells to which the term "reticular cell" can be unambiguously attached and it is probably better always to use the prefix "dendritic". These are the cells which though not highly phagocytic, retain antigen in sensitized lymphoid tissue germinal centres (Nossal et al., 1968a,b). Stuart and Davidson (1971a) have recently described stellate cells in tissue cultures of human lymph nodes as "reticular" cells. There is no evidence as to whether these are the same cells as have been given the name "reticular" cell in the intact body. The term "reticular cell" seems to be confusing and possibly redundant, and if used should be defined.

The term reticulum cell is even more difficult to interpret. Gall (1958) suggested that in any serious discussion of mesenchyme "the reticulum cell appears to be a myth". The term is used widely by histopathologists to describe a large cell with pale cytoplasm with few prominent inclusions and a large lepto-chromatic nucleus. It is inferred on morphological evidence that this is the cell from which a particular type of neoplasm, the reticulum cell sarcoma arises. The term should not be used to describe mature macrophages with numerous lysosomes and prominent cytoplasmic inclusions.

It is difficult to identify cells in normal rodent lymphoreticular tissues for which the term reticulum cell would be appropriate; in normal human lymphoid tissue however a small number of cells are present of irregular shape with many ribonucleoprotein particles in the cytoplasm but containing few lysosomes. These cells probably correspond to the "reticulum cell" of the light microscopist. There is no real agreement as to the origin or significance of these cells. They may be immature macrophages but more research is required into their origin and significance.

Another terminological problem which must be considered is the relationship between endothelial cells and macrophages. It seems reasonable to describe avidly phagocytic endothelial cells either as such or as "endothelial macrophages". The term "reticulo-endothelial cell", sometimes applied to these cells (Moore *et al.*, 1964), is sometimes used to describe all the cells of the RES and is ambiguous.

The various types of capillary endothelium have been classified by Bennett *et al.* (1959) according to the presence of fenestrae, the number of pinocytic vesicles and the patency of cell junctions; an exhaustive review of endothelial structure has been published by Majno (1964). It is clear that many endothelial cells will take up small amounts of colloid from the circulation after repeated administration of large doses (Cotran, 1965), but arbitrarily only those endothelial cells which take up large amounts of colloids are considered to belong to the reticuloendothelial system. Many earlier light microscopic reports on phagocytosis by endothelium have been ruled out by the demonstration by Majno and Palade (1961) that colloid may leak between endothelial cells after local injection of permeability factors. Both lymphatic endothelium and peritoneal mesothelium have considerable phagocytic power when large numbers of foreign particles are present (Casley-Smith, 1964, 1965).

Phagocytic endothelial cells are found in the liver, the spleen, bone marrow, the lymph sinuses of the lymph nodes and to a lesser extent in the post-capillary venules of lymph nodes and Peyer's patches.

In general such endothelial cells tend to be thicker than normal endothelium, with more processes, more vacuoles, and more dense bodies of varying types. There is in fact a continuous gradation of structure between non-phagocytic endothelial cells, moderately phagocytic endothelial cells and avidly phagocytic true macrophages.

When the doubtful and equivocal synonyms of "macrophage" have been considered the next problem is to give some sort of definition of the macrophage and to outline the approach to its study which will be followed in the rest of this text.

A macrophage is an avidly phagocytic metazoan cell with the cellular enzymes required to digest what it has ingested, and the cellular apparatus necessary to make more enzymes. It is found in two main forms, free and fixed. Free cells can wander throughout the tissues; fixed cells have a permanent, or at least semi-permanent settled site.

In the following chapters a description of the free macrophage will be followed by a description of the fixed macrophage. The origin and circulation of these cells will then be considered followed by a discussion of their behaviour in the artificial environment of tissue culture. Next the way in which macrophages ingest material from their environment will be discussed followed by a consideration of the way in which they act in the defence of the organism and its metabolism. The neoplasms of the macrophage and similar cells will be described, followed by a brief account of several cells which though not true macrophages, resemble the macrophage in varying degree. Most of the work that will be described relates to experimental animals; relatively little direct information exists on the human macrophage.

The Free Macrophage

Free macrophages occur scattered diffusely throughout the mammalian body; for present purposes free macrophages will be considered to be those which exist outside the major lymphoreticular organs. They fall into four major subdivisions: (a) the macrophages of the connective tissues or histiocytes; (b) the macrophages of serosal sacs; (c) the macrophages of inflammatory exudates; (d) the pulmonary alveolar macrophages. The first three of these groups will be considered together; alveolar macrophages which are rather distinct will be considered separately.

The classic accounts of the structure of the histiocyte are those of Maximow and his disciple, Bloom (Maximow and Bloom, 1931). The true histiocyte or resting wandering cell is a flat rounded oval or branched cell with an oval or kidney shaped nucleus smaller and denser than that of the fibroblast. A centriole and Golgi network were demonstrated by the early light microscopists as were mitochondria. Small granules or vacuoles in the cytoplasm stain with neutral red; the most characteristic feature of the cells is their ability to store colloidal dyes avidly, as opposed to fibroblasts which store little or no dye. Maximow and Bloom distinguished amoeboid active wandering cells varying in structure from a cell resembling "in every way the lymphocytes of the blood" to a large cell 12 μm in diameter "with an eccentric oval or kidney-shaped nucleus and highly amoeboid protoplasm containing various inclusions when stained supra-vitally with neutral red". Cells with these characteristics may be seen in connective tissues but the distinction between resting and amoeboid cells is probably not valid and it seems better to call them all histiocytes. These and other early authors describe morphological intermediates between a circulating lymphocytoid or monocytoid precursor, the "polyblast", and the histiocyte; and also between cells with pale staining (leptochromatic) nuclei and poorly defined cytoplasm, so-called primitive or undifferentiated mesenchymal cells, and histiocytes. The latter tissue precursor sometimes receives the title "reticular cell" a title which has been criticized and dismissed above. The evidence for the origin of macrophages in general will be discussed in a later chapter.

The serosal macrophages mainly derive ultimately from the bone marrow; they may come immediately from the subserosal lympho-reticular masses or milk spots (Ranvier, 1870) found both in peritoneum and in pleura. These are aggregates of lymphocytes and macrophages with a small blood vessel in the core, covered by mesothelial cells and true macrophages; the former are adherent to one another by desmosomes, the latter apparently not. Between the covering cells of the milk spots clefts pass down into the depths of the tissue, providing possible pathways for the entrance or exit of cells (Carr, 1967a).

The free cells in the serosal cavity are conveniently obtained by washing out the cavity with saline and have been a favourite subject for experiment (Cappell, 1929). The cells present include macrophages, lymphocytes, mast cells, mesothelial cells and a few neutrophil and eosinophil leucocytes. The exact proportions of these vary with species and with the mode of obtaining them. In the mouse, if some Hanks solution is injected after dislocating the animal's neck, and the fluid present in the abdominal cavity is removed after 2 min, it will be found to contain some 60% macrophages, 35% lymphoid cells and a residue of mast cells, eosinophils and degenerate mesothelial cells. In this species however, the percentage of mast cells in the peritoneal washout can vary very widely for no apparent reason. Moreover, if the cells present in the small amount of fluid actually lying in the peritoneal cavity are examined, a higher proportion of these will be found to be lymphoid. The number and proportion of cells present vary widely from species to species. The introduction of a stimulus several days before leads to the appearance of a fluid containing a high percentage of large mature macrophages.

Peritoneal macrophages are approximately spherical, and have a kidney-shaped nucleus with a prominent cytocentrum and neutral red granules (Maximow and Bloom, 1931). Granules staining with Romanowsky stains may also be seen (Cappell, 1929). In general bigger cells contain a larger number of stainable granules and often have a visibly irregular edge; such cells are notable in populations elicited by the injection of one or other irritant into the peritoneum. The number of cells which are classed as macrophages with the light microscope varies widely with species, experimental conditions and the personal vagaries of the observer. Even with the electron microscope cells often cannot be identified absolutely as lymphocyte or macrophage. Perkins *et al.* (1967) identified some 20% of cells in a normal population as macrophages by incubating them with opsonized RBC. On the other hand in a different strain of the same species about 60% or more of cells in a similarly normal population can be identified with the light microscope as phagocytosing carbon, and have the ultrastructural characteristics of macrophages (Carr, 1967a). Many of the general properties of mouse peritoneal macrophages were described and reviewed by Mims (1964a). He noted that some 1–3% of the cells labelled with tritiated thymidine and therefore were synthesizing DNA, and suggested that the length of life of a peritoneal macrophage might be about one week. Macrophages similar to those of the serosal cavities occur in the synovial cavities of joints.

The macrophages of inflammatory exudates morphologically resemble those of the serosal sacs but are very much more pleomorphic and contain much larger forms. Because of their importance in human pathology, they will be considered in detail in a later chapter.

Having differentiated these three groups initially, it should be emphasized that they are very similar; their cytochemistry and ultrastructure will be considered together.

The pulmonary alveolar macrophages differ in some respects from other free macrophages and will be considered separately.

Cytochemistry

Opie in 1906 showed that proteolytic enzymes were found in inflammatory lesions; macrophages have long been known to contain granules stainable with methylene blue eosin dye mixtures (e.g. Cappell, 1929). A correlation between these two observations is however only recent.

Acid phosphatase, the most readily demonstrable lysosomal enzyme, was shown to be present in large amounts in reticuloendothelial organs, and in inflammatory granulomata (Gomori, 1941; Barka *et al.*, 1961). There is some correlation between the content of acid phosphatase in the macrophages of a species and the resistance of that species to tuberculosis (Grogg and Pearse, 1952).

The wide range of enzymes since demonstrated in macrophages includes lipase, esterase of various types, β glucuronidase, β-galactosidase, lysozyme, cytochrome oxidase, peroxidase, naphthylamidase, acetyl glucosaminidase, ATPase, 5-nucleotidase and a variety of oxidative enzymes including succinate, lactate and malate dehydrogenases and NADP diaphorase (Monis *et al.*, 1968; Braunsteiner and Schmalzl, 1970 for review). Two distinct cathepsins with maximum activity at different pHs were identified by Stevanovic *et al.* (1962). Similarly Dannenberg and Bennett (1964) demonstrated two proteinases in rabbit mononuclear exudate cells, one like lung proteinase, the other like chymotrypsin. The field has recently been reviewed by Braunstein and Schmalzl (1970).

Day and his colleagues have carried out extensive biochemical investigations of macrophage esterases (see review by Day, 1964). Homogenates from rabbit peritoneal exudates can esterify cholesterol at pH 6·0 and hydrolyse cholesterol acetate at pH 7·3 but cannot hydrolyse cholesterol oleate. Moreover (Day, 1960) macrophages can oxidize chylomicron fat and unesterified fatty acids. The enzymes concerned have been identified as an esterase of the pseudo-cholinesterase type, and a lipase rather similar to pancreatic lipase (Day and Harris, 1960). It has been previously shown that broadly similar transformations can occur in living tissues after parenteral injection of various lipids (Day and French, 1959).

The enzyme content of macrophages varies with their physiological state. For instance during culture the acid phosphatase content of monocytes increases (Weiss and Fawcett, 1953; Goldstein and McCormick, 1957). Similarly after stimulation *in vivo* with attenuated tubercle bacilli (BCG) there is an increase in such enzymes as acid phosphatase, β-glucuronidase and lysozyme (Suter and Hulliger, 1960; Colwell and Hess, 1963; Myrvik *et al.*, 1962). Saito and Suter (1963) noted an increase in acid phosphatase, in β-glucuronidase and in cathepsin after intravenous injection of BCG, present both in free serosal macrophages, in liver homogenates and in plasma. These authors also noted that the acid phosphatase in cultured macrophages doubled in quantity in 24 hours, but that the β-glucuronidase content actually decreased in this time, a pointer that the behaviour of all lysosomal enzymes is not necessarily exactly parallel.

Dannenberg *et al.* (1963a, b) demonstrated clearly that stimulation of macrophages with particles led to an immediate increase in O_2 uptake, glucose consumption, CO_2 and lactic acid output, lipid turnover and phagocytic ability. They postulated an initial increase in motility and pseudopod formation; the cellular enzymes are not increased in amount, but used to capacity. They termed this protoplasmic excitation. Later they showed an increase in esterase and phosphatase and in digestive enzymes—protoplasmic adaptation.

The enzyme content of macrophages at different anatomical sites varies, possibly in relation to the varying degree of environmental stimulation at different sites. For instance the enzyme content of peritoneal cells was studied in detail by Cohn and Wiener (1963a, b) and compared with that of alveolar macrophages; β-glucuronidase, acid phosphatase, cathepsin, acid ribonuclease, lysozyme, esterase and lipase were identified and shown to be present on the whole in larger quantities in alveolar cells than in peritoneal cells. There was an increase in acid phosphatase, in lysozyme and in lipase in alveolar cells after stimulation by intratracheal injection of BCG. On ultracentrifugation of alveolar cells a large proportion of these hydrolytic enzymes was present in a lysosomal fraction composed of small granules sedimenting after 12 min at 15,000 **g,** and separable from mitochondria on a sucrose density gradient. These granules stained with neutral red and showed increased enzymatic activity after freezing.

The role of various hydrolytic enzymes in macrophage function is not always clear. For instance there is no good evidence as to just what is the function of acid phosphatase; useful suggestions have however been made about the function of other enzymes. For instance enzymes like galactosidase and aminopeptidase may hydrolyse the surface antigenic groups of bacteria ingested by the macrophages (Yarborough *et al.*, 1967). Lysozyme may hydrolyse the mucopolysaccharide framework of such organisms as the tubercle bacillus (Carson and Dannenberg, 1965). Ribonuclease and deoxyribonuclease hydrolyse the nucleoproteins of bacteria and of injured tissue. The deoxyribonuclease may release cationic antibacterial histones from nucleoproteins (Meyer *et al.*, 1970).

The chemistry and metabolism of macrophages was studied in detail by Oren *et al.* (1963). The respiratory activity of alveolar macrophages was high; that of the other phagocytes quite low. Both polymorphs and peritoneal macrophages convert most of their consumed glucose to lactate. The respiration of alveolar macrophages is stimulated by glucose while that of polymorphs and peritoneal macrophages is depressed. Lactate output increased in all types under anaerobic conditions; this was notably true of the alveolar macrophage.

The intracellular pH of macrophages was studied by Rous (1925a, b) using indicator dyes. Rous showed that the pH of the intracellular granules was 3·0 or less. Damaged cells did not segregate dye in this way, from which he inferred that "the healthy cell protects the acid reaction of intracellular granules", a forerunner of the lysosome concept. Sprick (1956) however again using indicator dyes found the pH-range of the intracellular granules to be 4·7 to 5·5. It seems likely at present that not too much reliance can be placed on experiments which depend on whether indicator dyes behave in precisely the same way in the complex intracellular milieu as they do under simpler conditions.

Ultrastructure

The ultrastructure of the peritoneal macrophage forms a convenient baseline for the description of the ultrastructure of macrophages in general. Later descriptions of macrophages in other sites will refer in the main to differences from the basic peritoneal type. Detailed accounts of the ultrastructure of peritoneal cells have been given by Tanaka (1958), North and Mackaness (1963a, b), Cohn et al. (1966a, b), Carr (1967a) and Dumont (1969), while briefer mention occurs in papers by e.g. Felix and Dalton (1956), Odor (1956) and Journey (1963).

As seen in a transmission electron micrograph peritoneal macrophages are circular or nearly so in outline, that is their form in three dimensions is near to spherical. The cell surface is however irregular; small processes or pseudopodia project from it. Some of these are clearly finger-like, showing a circular cross-section while others are flap-like. The larger of these processes are often flattened back against the surface of the cell whether artefactually or in reality, and enclose cleft-like spaces. In addition there are numerous deep almost spherical indentations of the surface 0·1 μm or more in diameter which give the appearance of vacuoles (Fig. 1).

The scanning electron microscope gives a striking view of the external surface of the macrophage, though current specimen preparation techniques are fraught with the hazard of artefact. The cells vary from spherical in shape according to the degree of stimulation they have undergone. Ridge-like elevations cover the more mature cells, presumably corresponding to the ruffles seen in fresh preparations. Larger flap-like processes may also be seen, possibly corresponding to the hyaloplasmic veils seen in moving cells (Carr *et al.*, 1969) (Figs 2 and 3).

In transmission micrographs the surface membrane shows the usual three layered appearance. The membrane has quite well marked nucleoside phosphatase activity (North, 1966a).

When the cells are stained with semi-specific stains for acid mucopolysaccharides a very prominent cell coat is displayed (Curran *et al.*, 1966; Carr *et al.*, 1970). This is best seen after ruthenium red staining as an amorphous layer 8–16 nm thick with occasional areas of poorly defined fibrillar appearance. It is apparently adherent to the outer layer of the unit membrane from which it cannot be clearly differentiated. Masses of electron dense material of similar appearance may be scattered over the surface of the coat and fine strands of similar material cross indentations on the cell surface. The coat is not readily digested by enzymes but is presumably composed largely of acidic mucosubstances. It may be of importance in such phenomena as recognition of foreign material, phagocytosis and adhesion to glass surfaces (Fig. 7).

Flask-shaped caveolae or indentations occur infrequently on the cell surface and contain densely staining material having the same appearance as the cell coat. There is no increase in the number of these caveolae when pinocytosis is stimulated; these caveolae may conceivably represent the mechanism whereby the macrophage secretes its coat substance (Carr *et al.*, 1970). Deep "worm-like" invaginations of the cell surface, containing cell coat material, have been demonstrated in guinea-pig macrophages (Brederoo and Daems, 1972).

The membrane systems of the macrophage are well developed. The granular endoplasmic reticulum is prominent in peritoneal as in other macrophages. It is comprised as is usual of channels whose membranes are studded on the cytoplasmic side by ribosomes. It commonly forms a shell near the cell surface within which lie the Golgi zone, cell centre and developing granules. Granular endoplasmic reticulum is best developed in large mature macrophages. The Golgi zone is prominent particularly in large mature macrophages, and is composed of elongated flattened cisterns and small vesicles. In this region occasional areas of junction between smooth and rough endoplasmic reticulum may be seen (Figs 4 and 5.)

Numerous other membranous elements are present in macrophage cytoplasm but their significance is not always clear. Many apparent vacuoles some 0·5 μm to 1 μm in diameter lie near the surface probably representing merely deep surface invaginations. Scattered more deeply in the cytoplasm of normal peritoneal macrophages are smaller smooth-surfaced vesicles 50–100 nm in diameter, prominent in the Golgi zone and also immediately below the cell surface. In culture these vesicles may be seen to fuse with larger vesicles (Hirsch *et al.*, 1968). Small cytoplasmic vesicles have been described as fusing with phagocytic vacuoles and being by inference primary lysosomes (North and Mackaness, 1963b). The contents of many of these vesicles stain positively with uranyl acetate; such vesicles therefore appear in material so treated to have electron dense cores. Small vesicles containing electron-dense material and associated channels or short tubular profiles often containing electron-dense material have been interpreted as smooth endoplasmic reticulum and may represent stages in lysosome synthesis.

Also present in peritoneal macrophage cytoplasm are variable numbers of coated vesicles best seen in stimulated mature macrophages (Carr, 1968a; Dumont, 1969). These vesicles are surrounded by a coat of small radiating bristles, 20 nm long. Such vesicles have been noted in such varied sites as the mosquito oöcyte (Roth and Porter, 1964) and rat vas deferens (Friend and Farquar, 1967) to be associated with the absorption of protein into cells.

In addition where peritoneal cells are cultured in media containing high concentrations of protein there is a regular flow of pinocytic vacuoles into them as shown by electron-dense markers. These vacuoles measure $0 \cdot 1$ μm or more in diameter (Cohn *et al.*, 1966). It is not certain to what extent this happens *in vivo*. Very large vacuoles appear in macrophages treated with chloroquine and have been interpreted as autophagic vacuoles (Fedorko *et al.*, 1968a, b), and therefore presumably suggest cellular degeneration.

The presence of electron dense granules in peritoneal macrophages was first pointed out by Tanaka (1958). These electron-dense granules are probably the same as the granules staining with Romanowsky stains depicted by Cappell (1929) in peritoneal macrophages and are akin to the azurophil granules of monocytes. Similar structures were described by North and Mackaness (1963a) as vesicles with dense staining material and contained acid phosphatase (North, 1966b; Carr, 1968a). These granules have a consistent sometimes ordered fine structure, showing conspicuous densities in the 8–10 nm range and around 3 nm, though there may well be a continuous spectrum of sizes (Figs 8 and 9). These densities are best seen in sections stained with uranyl and lead salts; they may represent aggregates of hydrolytic enzyme or alternatively masses of non-ferritin iron. Ferritin may be present, though much less commonly in peritoneal macrophages than in those from other sites. Macrophages can synthesize ferritin from inorganic iron, though the ultrastructural mechanism of this has not been fully explored (Richter, 1959; Muir and Golberg, 1961a, b). The larger granules contain varying amounts of lipids, often in lamellar form. After stimulation with lipid emulsions large granules appear which contain lipid. Similarly after macrophages were stimulated to pinocytosis *in vitro* the large dense bodies were shown to incorporate labelled lysine and marker particles (Cohn and Benson, 1965a, b, c; Cohn *et al.*, 1966a, b.)

These granules are quite characteristic of macrophages and are probably mostly lysosomes. It is nevertheless clear that only rarely do all the granules in a cell give a positive acid phosphatase reaction (Fig. 6). It seems likely that some of them may contain peroxidase. The larger hetero-geneous granules are clearly secondary or mixed lysosomes. The smaller homogeneous granules are probably primary lysosomes (Carr, 1968a). This view is supported by the presence of similar granules in macrophages elsewhere: in splenic and lymph node macrophages and histiocytes (Kaji-kawa, 1964; Onoe and Tsukada, 1964) and indeed throughout the RES (Carr, 1968b), in studies of the effects of silica on macrophages (Allison *et al.*, 1966) and in tuberculous granulomata (Dumont and Sheldon, 1965; Galindo and Imaeda, 1966). Similar small granules in lung macrophages have been shown to fuse with vesicles containing ingested material and to be by inference primary lysosomes (Leake and Myrvik, 1966, 1968, 1970). Small azurophil granules have been shown to occur in circulating mono-cytes. These are similar in structure to the smallest granules in peritoneal macrophages (Nichols *et al.*, 1971).

Dumont (1969) in a study of the maturation *in vivo* of hamster peritoneal macrophages has however pointed out that it is not always possible to characterize the previous history of a lysosomal granule in a peritoneal macrophage from its structure. This author also was unable to follow sequentially previous reported pathways of lysosome formation and found an acid phosphatase reaction only in Golgi vesicles and relatively large lysosomes.

It seems reasonable at present to suppose that the smaller homogeneous dense bodies in electron micrographs of macrophages stained with uranium and lead salts represent primary lysosomes. Further work on the ultra-structural cytochemistry of macrophages is required.

The ultrastructural mechanism of the motility of the macrophages is not clear. Bundles of microfibrils about 5 nm in diameter were first demonstrated in the cytoplasm of monocytes by de Petris *et al.* (1962), and have subsequently been shown to occur in macrophages in many other sites including the peritoneum. These microfibrils are of the right dimensions to be actin fibrils, and may be contractile (Allison *et al.*, 1971.)

Microtubules some 20 nm in diameter also occur in peritoneal macrophages commonly radiating from the usually paired centrioles. The function of these is unknown but may be skeletal. Long membranous channels were described by North and Mackaness (1963a) as being possibly related to cell movement. It now seems likely that these represent fixation artefacts.

The mitochondria of peritoneal macrophages are generally elongated, 1–4 μm in length with the usual shelf-like cristae and mitochondrial granules, and are in general unremarkable. There are occasionally a few small lipid globules in the cytoplasm. Free ribonucleoprotein granules are found scattered through the cytoplasmic sap. These are rather more frequent and more often aggregated into polysomes in larger mature macrophages. The ectoplasmic area beneath the cell membrane is well developed and at high resolution contains small granules and occasional fine fibrils.

The nucleus is usually indented especially in more mature cells. It shows conventional nuclear structure—nucleopores are prominent, the lamina densa below the nuclear membrane is well formed and the chromatin usually shows related perichromatin and interchromatin granules. A nucleolus with RNP granules and associated chromatin is often seen.

A number of interesting changes occur, when peritoneal macrophages are stimulated in various ways, either simply by growing *in vitro* in a culture medium or with substances such as lipopolysaccharide (Cohn and Benson, 1965a, b, c) or glycerol trioleate (Carr, 1967b, 1968a; Carr and Williams, 1967). The cells enlarge and form more dense granules or lysosomes (Cohn and Benson, 1965; Cohn *et al.*, 1966a, b; Carr, 1968a). Pinocytosis plays a significant but not fully understood part in this. Dense material is found within the endoplasmic reticulum of stimulated cells which is similar to that forming the substance of small dense bodies.

Peritoneal macrophages stimulated with *Listeria monocytogenes* were shown by Blanden (1968) to have more lysosomes than normal cells and to be more active in destroying bacteria, though phagocytosis does not seem to be more rapid. The more rapid destruction may be related to the high content of hydrolytic enzymes. Dense material similar to that seen in lysosomes can be seen in phagocytic vacuoles after phagocytosis (Wiener *et al.*, 1965; Carr, 1968b; Blanden, 1968) (Fig. 19).

When peritoneal macrophages are stimulated with triglyceride emulsions they contain numerous large heterogeneous dense bodies which are obviously residual bodies or mixed lysosomes (Carr, 1968a). In peritoneal macrophages from animals injected with ascites tumour cells, large tubular elements occur in lysosome-like bodies; the nature of these is obscure (Journey, 1963).

With certain particulate stimuli, e.g. glycerol trioleate or glucan *in vitro* or *in vivo*, the cytoplasmic processes of the cells (both flap-like and finger-like) become elongated (Carr, 1967b, 1968a) (Fig. 10). When stimulated cells were examined with the scanning electron microscope they were found to have more prominent flap-like processes than normal cells, and in addition to have large flange-like processes. This may be due to an increase in the deformability of the whole cell (Carr *et al.*, 1968). Similar changes have been demonstrated by Albrecht *et al.* (1972). These changes are probably associated with an increase in phagocytic ability (Cooper and West, 1964; Carr, 1967b). When tritiated triglycerides were used to stimulate the cells, it was found by EM autoradiography that the areas where membrane stimulation was obvious had numerous associated autoradiographic grains (Williams and Carr, 1968). Similar surface changes can be induced in polymorphs with such particulate stimulants as bacteria (Lockwood and Allison, 1966) in blood monocytes by stimulation with mycoplasma (Zucker-Franklin *et al.*, 1966) and in pulmonary alveolar macrophages by stimulation with BCG (Leake and Myrvik, 1968); the surface effect of these stimulants may be related merely to particle size and charge. A similar protrusion of pseudopodia occurs when macrophages are heavily irradiated or treated with lysolecithin. It may therefore under some circumstances be a degenerative or predegenerative phenomenon (Wilkinson and Cater, 1969; Sanders and Adee, 1969). This non-specific stimulation may be different from the more specific processes involved in the production of the "immune macrophage" (North and Mackaness, 1963b); after injection of *Listeria monocytogenes* the peritoneal cells have fewer processes, and a denser cytoplasmic matrix than normal. These cells have an increased ability to phagocytose *Listeria* (North and Mackaness, 1963b). Blanden (1968) showed a marked increase in lysosomes after similar stimulation. Hard (1969) found that "immune" macrophages had smoother surfaces than normal. Five days after stimulation with Freund's adjuvant the macrophages present in the rat peritoneal cavity have smoother surfaces and are rounder than normal (Mayhew and Williams, 1971).

Non-specific stimulation of macrophages in fact induces a maturation of the macrophage from a small cell with few small processes and little digestive enzyme, to a large cell with longer processes, more digestive enzyme and more phagocytic ability. It seems however that increase in cell roughness may sometimes be only a transient phenomenon and that cells may thereafter round up—whether in degeneration or because of exhaustion of membrane. A comparable process may occur throughout the RES and may account in part for increases in RE clearance (Carr, 1967). A similar reaction of peritoneal macrophages to tumour cells may be associated with inhibition of tumour growth (Ito and Miura, 1966). A similar process of maturation occurs when monocytes are cultivated *in vitro* (Sutton and Weiss, 1965; Cohn *et al.*, 1966a, b; Sutton, 1967) and may account for the formation of the large macrophages commonly seen in chronic inflammatory lesions.

The subcutaneous tissue histiocyte is rather similar to the peritoneal macrophage (Kajikawa, 1964; Kajikawa *et al.*, 1970) (Fig. 11). Various stages in maturation can be seen; commonly the smooth endoplasmic reticulum and Golgi zone are well-developed and the vesicles of the endoplasmic reticulum may contain material similar to that of the mature lysosomes or H-granules (Kajikawa, 1964). These are membrane-bound with an electron-dense core and may show myelin-like structure. After the injection of silver proteinate, particles were not seen in the H-granules, which were therefore regarded as primary lysosomes. These cells also contained phagosomes—membrane-bound vesicles containing phagocytosed material (e.g. silver proteinate particles) and amorphous material. The findings of Yamori and Mori (1964) were similar; after injections of egg albumen or tubercle bacilli cells appeared whose cytoplasm was more electron dense and which contained more cytoplasmic RNP particles and sometimes well developed granular endoplasmic reticulum. The cell illustrated (Fig. 11) is a rather small histiocyte.

Similar descriptions are given of macrophages in the lamina propria of the gut (Deane, 1964) and in the pulp of the tooth (Han and Avery, 1965). A similar account was given by Goldberg *et al.* (1962) of histiocytes in a delayed hypersensitivity reaction. Histiocytes were noted (Wiener *et al.*, 1965) to have markedly ruffled borders, compared with other cells in inflammatory lesions and to have prominent cytoplasmic membrane systems.

By contrast Gieseking (1963) believed that histiocytes could be distinguished from fibroblasts by the paucity of their endoplasmic reticulum and suggested that their granules were merely phagocytosed inclusions. The latter view of histiocyte inclusions was also taken by Deane (1964) and Han and Avery (1965). It must be emphasized that while many macrophage inclusions are of this nature, the similarity of some of the smaller dense bodies to the azurophil granules of myelocytes is very strong evidence of their secretory nature.

Pulmonary Alveolar Macrophages

In pulmonary tissue, cells which look rather like macrophages elsewhere may be found (1) in the interstitial connective tissue of the alveolar wall (2) forming part of the lining epithelium of the alveolus, the great alveolar cells of Sorokin (1966) (3) free in the lumen of the alveolus. Some of the latter are true macrophages and others are free shed greater alveolar cells.

An understanding of the pulmonary macrophages depends on some knowledge of the structure of the alveolar wall. This has been extensively reviewed by Bertalanaffy (1964a, b) to whose papers reference may be made for the early literature. Apart from the thin epithelial cells lining the alveoli, numerous cuboidal cells may be seen often wedged in an angle of the alveolus. These may be 20 μm or more in diameter; some are vacuolated and contain sudanophilic lipid and cholesterol, and are of epithelial origin—the great alveolar epithelial cells. Others, less vacuolated and containing less lipid are true macrophages and are much more phagocytic than the great alveolar cells. The free cells found in the lumen of the alveoli are mainly but not entirely true macrophages. From the alveolar lumen some of the cells are reabsorbed by lymphatics but most actively migrate into the bronchioles, find their way onto the carpet of mucus and are wafted up by ciliary action. The alveolar phagocytes may contain haemosiderin pigment (in cardiac failure) or carbon dust, and are then called "heart-failure cells" and "dust cells" respectively (Fig. 12).

The origin of the free alveolar phagocytes has for long been the subject of debate. This problem is discussed in Chapter Five; it is clear that many alveolar macrophages may be of marrow origin, and some derive from mesenchymal cells in the alveolar septa. Some others may derive from the great alveolar epithelial cells, the structure of which is considered in a later chapter.

The fine structure of the free alveolar macrophages was described by Low (1952), Schulz (1959) and Karrer (1958, 1960). These cells contain a moderate amount of smooth endoplasmic reticulum and relatively little rough endoplasmic reticulum. They have numerous processes and invaginations at their surfaces. Many inclusion bodies or lysosomes are present, often containing myelin figures or ferritin. Occasionally these structures are paracrystalline. Alveolar macrophages are larger than the peritoneal macrophages of the same species, with less endoplasmic reticulum and Golgi membranes, but more lysosomes. Their mitochondria are rounder though not larger (Leake and Heise, 1967) but are probably more numerous.

Marked accumulation and differentiation of pulmonary alveolar macrophages can be induced by the intravenous administration of BCG. There is a progressive increase in endoplasmic reticulum and dense bodies in these cells accompanied by a correlated increase in the lysozyme content of the serum of the animals, and in cell-free extracts of the cells. The cells with more endoplasmic reticulum and more granules had notably more pseudopodia (Leake and Myrvik, 1968).

Some information as to the origin of alveolar macrophages has been obtained by electron microscopy. Macrophages and mesenchymal cells which contain lipid are found in the connective tissue of the alveolar septa. Moreover after intravenous stimulation of Freund's adjuvant, mitosis was seen in monocytes in pulmonary capillaries (Galindo and Imaeda, 1966). A sequence has been traced between small monocytoid cells and macrophages in populations of cells washed out of alveoli (Policard et al., 1963). These findings support the idea that in the main alveolar macrophages are of mesenchymal and ultimately marrow origin. The presence of some osmiophilic masses in free alveolar cells which otherwise look like typical macrophages could be interpreted as due to secondary ingestion of masses of surfactant derived from great alveolar cells but more likely means that some free alveolar macrophages derive from great alveolar epithelial cells.

Whatever their precise origin an interesting population of cells can be obtained by washing out rabbit lungs in an atraumatic fashion (Myrvik et al., 1961a). Most of the cells obtained were actively phagocytic cells having rather more similarity in appearance to plasma cells than most phagocytes. These cells were fairly resistant to osmotic shock, resisting 0·2% NaCl for 15 min at 25 °C, and did not show evidence of multiplication in culture. They contained very much more lysozyme than peritoneal cells (Myrvik et al., 1961b). A two-fold increase in the yield of cells with a higher lysozyme content was produced four days after a single intravenous dose of BCG vaccine. If the intravenous dose followed on prior subcutaneous vaccination with BCG, the cellular response was very extensive and the cells more heterogeneous than normal. They contained however less lysozyme than normal, possibly because they came from the marrow or some other extra-pulmonary source (Myrvik et al., 1962).

Heise and Myrvik (1967) showed that rabbit alveolar macrophages cultivated *in vitro* secreted lysozyme and to a lesser extent acid phosphatase and cathepsin into the medium; secretion was inhibited by inhibitors of protein synthesis.

Mouse alveolar cells were studied by Cohn and Wiener (1963) and shown to contain more β-glucuronidase, acid phosphatase, cathepsin, acid ribonuclease, lysozyme, esterase and lipase than their peritoneal counterparts. BCG vaccination produced an increase in the acid phosphatase, lysozyme and lipase content of the alveolar cells. Goggins *et al.* (1968) have demonstrated hyaluronidase in rabbit alveolar macrophages.

It is necessary to be slightly wary of these studies of "alveolar macrophages" washed out in this way. Moore *et al.* (1964a) showed that after intravenous injection of Freund's adjuvant a gross increase occurred in the number of cells in the alveoli. These originated initially from circulating monocytes and later by proliferation of mesenchymal cells in the alveolar walls. Late in the reaction numerous epithelial cells could be distinguished in the alveoli with the electron microscope; light microscopically however they could not be distinguished from macrophages. Alveolar macrophages obtained by lung washout may therefore be rather impure preparations. An interesting feature of this reaction (Moore *et al.*, 1964b) was the presence of γ-globulin in many of the macrophages, when the animals were injected with Freund's adjuvant and diphtheria toxoid. Some of this globulin was undoubtedly specific antibody.

Chapter Two

THE FIXED MACROPHAGES

These occur in the liver, the spleen, bone marrow, the lymph nodes, in the central nervous system (microglia), and in the placenta.

Kupffer Cells

The "*sternzellen*" or stellate cells of the liver were first described by von Kupffer using a gold chloride impregnation technique (1876). The early work has been reviewed by Aterman (1963). The original illustration by von Kupffer of a stellate cell with many thin cytoplasmic processes is now usually regarded as an artefact, due to contraction and distortion of the cell induced by toxic fluids. Clearly as illustrated both in the earlier literature and by Aterman (1963) in freeze-dried materials there are two kinds of cell. One is larger than the other and bulges further into the lumen, often assuming a rather triangular or wedge-shaped appearance, sometimes with processes which cross the lumen. These, the Kupffer cells, are more actively phagocytic than endothelial cells; they are on the whole more numerous at the periphery of liver lobules (Lison and Smulders, 1948; Howard, 1959). From the extensive literature on the structure of Kupffer cells as seen by light microscopy (reviewed by Aterman, 1963), it is clear that Kupffer cells can on the whole be distinguished from endothelial cells by their larger nuclei and more prominent mitochondria and Golgi apparatus.

The cytochemistry of the Kupffer cell has been reviewed by Wachstein (1963). In general the resolution in light microscopic cytochemical studies is not great enough to allow clear distinction between endothelial cell and Kupffer cell. It is now well established that in most species there are small but variable amounts of glycoprotein, staining by the periodic acid Schiff (PAS) technique, and probably lysosomal. This material increases in several kinds of liver damage, and dramatically in haemolytic anaemia. Similar material appears in araldite sections to stain with toluidine blue. In some species Kupffer cells contain histochemically demonstrable lipid and RNA (Novikoff and Essner, 1960).

In the unstimulated state acid phosphatase, various non-specific esterases, deoxyribonuclease and glucuronidase may be demonstrated in Kupffer cells (Gomori, 1941; Wachstein, 1963). Wachstein (1963) suggests that "acid phosphatase and to a lesser degree esterase reflect to some extent the functional state of the RE cells in the liver".

After stimulation in various ways morphological changes occur in the Kupffer cells. A wide variety of stimuli induce an increase in the number and size of phagocytic cells, varying with the species. Such stimuli include splenectomy and injections of various metal salts and even dextrose. There is an increase in PAS positive glycoprotein (Wachstein, 1963) and in acid phosphatase (Howard, 1959; Jenkin and Benacerraf, 1960; Thorbecke et al., 1963) after widely varying stimuli. After stimulation with glucan there is a gross proliferation of phagocytic cells in the hepatic sinusoids. (Riggi and Diluzio, 1961; Ashworth et al., 1963).

An interesting comparison between methods of producing experimental hyperplasia of reticulo-endothelial cells was provided by Machado et al. (1968). The administration to rats of dimethylaminoazobenzene induced haemolytic anaemia and the excess red cell products released induced hyperplasia (Lozzio, 1967) of endothelial cells and macrophages in liver and spleen. The hyperplastic cells showed an increase in acid phosphatase and non-specific esterase, in PAS positive material and in iron storage. A similar proliferation occurring after injection of zymosan developed into nodular aggregates, while after injection of methyl cellulose there was grossly nodular accumulation of macrophages containing the foreign material, leading to marked distortion of the reticulin framework. It seems likely that nodular aggregation of macrophages results from the accumulation of excessive amounts of indigestible material.

Such stimulation of Kupffer cells is often accompanied by an increase in the rapidity with which colloids are cleared from the blood stream. This is easy to understand when the number of phagocytic cells is increased, as after glucan stimulation. After stimulation with glycerol trioleate emulsions (Stuart et al., 1960) there is no such increase in the number of cells and it is possible that the phagocytes may have increased surface activity as manifested by more or longer processes. Reduction in Kupffer cell function may under various circumstances be related to degenerative changes in the cells (Stuart, 1962) or blockage of the surface adhesion phase of phagocytosis (Wiener *et al.*, 1967). On repeated stimulation it appears at the light microscope level that most of the endothelial cells of the liver become highly phagocytic Kupffer cells (Bailiff, 1963).

Ultrastructure

The avid phagocytic properties of the cells lining hepatic sinusoids early attacted the attention of the electron microscopist (Parks and Chiquoine, 1957; Hampton, 1958). The fine structure of the Kupffer cell and of the hepatic sinusoid has been extensively reviewed by Rouiller and Jezequel (1963) and Aterman (1963). As pointed out by Kuhn and Oliver (1965) the structure of hepatic sinusoids varies with functional and nutritional state, from one species to another (Wood, 1963), and from one point to another in the liver lobule (Burkel and Low, 1965). The structure of the sinusoid of the rat liver is clearly described by Burkel and Low (1965). The peripheral part of the sinusoid has a continuous endothelial lining with an underlying basement membrane. In the intermediate part (90% of the length of the sinusoid) gaps are present between adjacent endothelial cells. Such gaps may vary due to contraction of adjacent cells. The short centrilobular portion resembles the peripheral part. Rather similar patterns exist in other species (Hampton, 1964). Adjacent endothelial cells may be bound to one another by desmosomes, whereas Kupffer cells are not held together by desmosomes; moreover the basement membrane present deep to endothelial cells is often defective below Kupffer cells. The endothelial lining of the sinusoid is interrupted in some species but not others (Casley-Smith and Read, 1965; Carstein, 1961; Karrer, 1961).

Accounts of the constituent cells of the wall of the sinusoid vary. Most authors describe the existence of two cell types, the endothelial cell and Kupffer cell though varying in their view as to whether these are totally distinct types. Among other workers Yamagishi (1959) and Carstein (1961) put forward the view that the cell types were totally distinct; this view has recently and compellingly been stated by Wisse (1970, 1972).

The Kupffer cell (Fig. 13) (Yamagishi, 1959; Schmidt, 1960; Burkel and Low, 1965; Wisse and Daems, 1970) is a bulky cell which often protrudes far into the sinusoid. The nucleocytoplasmic ratio is relatively low and the surface is highly differentiated showing numerous finger-like and flap-like pseudopodia, usually individually fairly short in unstimulated animals. These become prominent and probably longer during phagocytosis or

average endothelial cells, but not nearly so phagocytic as macrophages.

These endothelial cells contain prominent aggregates of microfibrils, interspersed with small granules, probably RNP granules. The whole aggregate stains densely with uranyl acetate (Weiss, 1957). These microfibrils may be related to the fact that the sinus endothelial cells are known to undergo active contraction. The endothelial cells are closely apposed but separate where blood cells pass through the wall (Figs 16 and 17). Deep to these lies an incomplete basement membrane, on the outside surface of which in some species is a row of fibroblasts. In the intersinusoidal tissue are found lymphocytes, macrophages and red and white blood cells; arterioles lying in the intersinusoidal tissue did not seem to connect directly with sinusoids. While some collapsed sinusoids are found in the intersinusoidal tissue of the red pulp, the intersinusoidal tissue is not in general composed of collapsed sinusoids (Moore et al., 1964; Simon and Pictet, 1964).

The white pulp of the spleen is merely a lymphoid tissue composed of a few fibroblasts and scanty collagen framework, many lymphocytes and a few macrophages.

The fine structure of the splenic macrophage has been studied by Weiss (1957) and Moore (1964) and by Galindo and Imaeda (1964); Thomas (1967); Daems and Persijn (1964); Roberts and Latta (1964); and recently in detail by Burke and Simon (1970a, b); and Simon and Burke (1970). The latter authors describe "reticulum cells" as cells larger than lymphocytes with more cytoplasm and organelles, and possessing some rough endoplasmic reticulum and free ribosomes. Some of these cells were stellate with long cytoplasmic prolongations; those which contained obvious phagocytic debris were termed macrophages. While most splenic macrophages lie in the red pulp, there are some in the white pulp. All have a similar structure (Weiss, 1964; Galindo and Imaeda, 1962; Sakuma, 1966) and here will be considered together. Many of the terminal arterial capillaries in some species, e.g. the dog are "sheathed" by macrophages of similar structure to those elsewhere in the spleen (Weiss, 1962; Zwillenberg and Zwillenberg, 1962).

The splenic macrophage tends to have rather more processes than macrophages in many sites; those which are most phagocytic tend to have most processes. These often interdigitate (Pictet et al., 1969a). As usual in macrophages there is a fairly prominent granular endoplasmic reticulum often showing Y-shaped branchings (Galindo and Imaeda, 1962); vesicles and membranous channels of various sizes are seen and the Golgi zone is often distinct. Microfibrils and microtubules are usually obvious, the former often in small bundles. The striking thing however about the splenic macrophage is the presence of numerous prominent lysosomes. Some of these are small and homogeneous and are probably primary lysosomes, but most are larger, sometimes 2–3 μm in diameter and heterogeneous in structure, containing fragments of red blood cells in various stages of disintegration, ferritin and myelin figures. It is possible that prior to ingestion by macrophages the older and more fragile red blood cells are mechanically damaged by being squeezed between the lining cells of the sinusoids to enter the cord spaces. In many species (notably the mouse) macrophages may contain ingested lymphocytes in various stages of disintegration—the so called tingible bodies (Swartzendruber and Congdon, 1963) (Figs 18 and 19). In the rat spleen some macrophages are found surrounded by clusters of mature red blood cells, presumably old red blood cells undergoing phagocytosis, while others are surrounded by or actually contain erythroblasts. Pictet *et al.* (1969b) postulate that the macrophages may be acting as nurse cells for the erythroblasts, somehow facilitating their maturation.

Splenic macrophages phagocytose intravenously injected carbon very rapidly (within 30 seconds of injection) by pushing pseudopods between endothelial cells into the lumen of sinusoids. It is probable that blood platelets play an important part in trapping particles for presentation to the macrophages (Burke and Simon, 1970b). Edwards and Simon (1970) studied red cell destruction in rat spleen and showed that in the red pulp and adjacent parts of the white pulp whole red cells were ingested by macrophages but not by endothelial cells. The ingested red blood cell loses its homogeneous structure and becomes heterogeneous and granular. The membrane of the phagosome becomes inverted in a complex way into the red cell and degenerate remnants of red cell come to lie in a complex set of tunnels ("tunnelization"). Ferritin particles collect along the margins of the inclusion just below the membrane, and then appear to penetrate the membrane into the adjacent cytoplasm. Although the term "reticular cell" is sometimes used to infer a phagocytic cell which lays down reticulin, there is no good evidence that one cell type can be responsible for both phagocytosis and deposition of reticulin or collagen (Moore *et al.*, 1964; Pictet *et al.*, 1969a).

Marrow Macrophages

Since early investigations on the uptake of injected particles from the circulation it has been known that some cells in the red bone marrow could sequestrate foreign material (see Hudson and Yoffey, 1963 for full references to the early literature). It is clear that to some extent and to a degree varying from species to species both the endothelial cells and the parenchymal macrophages of the marrow are actively phagocytic. However, much of the earlier work in this field was vitiated by the fact that the particles injected were themselves sufficiently toxic to produce increased vascular permeability.

Hudson and Yoffey (1963) investigated the problem in the guinea-pig using shellac-free and non-toxic carbon suspensions. It was found that carbon was seen initially in endothelial cells and after about an hour in parenchymal macrophages; large quantities accumulated in the parenchymal cells but occasional particles were seen in the endothelium even at one month after injection. A rather similar picture was noted by Hashimoto (1966). While endothelium contained some esterase and acid phosphatase, parenchymal macrophages showed no cytochemically demonstrable esterase but considerable amounts of acid phosphatase.

The ultrastructure of red bone marrow has been investigated by Pease (1956), Zamboni and Pease (1961) Weiss (1961, 1962, 1965) and Huhn (1966). The sinusoids are lined by flattened endothelial cells, poor in cytoplasmic organelles and held together by desmosomes. Gaps exist between the endothelial cell in some species but not in some others (Lindblad and Bjorkman, 1964). Outside the endothelium is an incomplete basement membrane, and outside that again adventitial cells, some of which at least are macrophages; other macrophages lie between the sinusoids. When intravenous colloids are given to experimental animals the particles are sometimes taken up by the endothelial cells and sometimes pass between the endothelial cells and are phagocytosed by interstitial macrophages. Just which pathway is followed seems to depend on the degree of increased vascular permeability excited by the colloid, i.e. on its toxicity (Weiss, 1961; Huhn and Steidle, 1967; Hudson and Yoffey, 1968).

Characteristically the marrow macrophage is found lying in the centre of a group of erythroblasts, forming a so-called erythroblastic islet. Numerous cytoplasmic processes pass out between the erythroblasts but there are relatively few phagocytic or pinocytic vesicles as compared with macrophages at other sites. Similarly granular endoplasmic reticulum is rather poorly developed. The conspicuous feature of the cytoplasm is the presence of numerous large pleomorphic secondary lysosomes, some clearly composed of degenerate red blood cells. Both these and the surrounding cytoplasm contain large quantities of ferritin (Figs 20 and 21). Bessis and

Breton Gorius (1959) claimed that iron in the form of ferritin was transferred from the macrophages to adjacent erythroblasts; Berman (1967) suggested that there were too few pinocytic vesicles at the edge of the macrophages for this to be likely. In aged mice striking crystalloids of unknown composition and significance occur; these are encrusted at their edges with ferritin (Berman, 1967; Hudson, 1968, 1969). Considerable amounts of acid phosphatase are present in the lysosomes of marrow macrophages (Kawabata and Azakawa, 1965).

There is a divergence of opinion as to whether the sinusoidal endothelial cells and the interstitial macrophages are fundamentally different cells. Weiss (1965) postulated that in haemolytic anaemia the sinusoidal lining cells could readily turn into cords of macrophages. Watanabe (1965) on the other hand showed that after irradiation of bone marrow the endothelium of the sinusoids was thicker than normal, with more desmosomes and thicker basement membrane; there was moreover an interstitial proliferation of "reticulum" cells, presumably immature macrophages. He believed this to be evidence of the fundamental difference between these cells. After this trauma pseudopodial processes of parenchymal macrophages sometimes protruded into the sinusoids, between endothelial cells.

Lymph Node Macrophages

The structure of the lymph node is well described in the earlier editions of Maximow and Bloom's textbook (1931) and by Drinker and Yoffey (1941). Lymph flows into a bowl-shaped subcapsular sinus crossed by fibrous trabeculae and blood vessels, and by a fine meshwork of cellular processes. The walls of the sinuses are formed by "reticulo-endothelial" cells and not by lining endothelium and tend to be incomplete where lymphatic growth is active. They are thus more complete in the medullary region. When carbon is perfused through a node at physiological pressures it is taken up both by the cells lining the sinuses and by extrasinusoidal macrophages. Carbon suspensions when used as a stain for fixed tissues *in vitro* outline circumferential cells round the edge of the follicle (Menzies, 1965).

The components of the lymph node have further been studied by silver staining and by enzyme cytochemical techniques. Marshall (1956) demonstrated metalophil cells lining the sinusoids; he designated these as syncytial, though this would not now be accepted. Solitary metalophil cells are scattered throughout the medulla.

Gomori (1941) drew attention to the presence of acid phosphatase in lymph nodes. Braunstein *et al.* (1958) studied human lymph nodes cytochemically in some detail. The cells lining the sinuses and the macrophages around the lymphoid follicles contained esterase, acid phosphatase and some phosphamidase. In addition cells were present in the germinal centres which did not react for these enzymes but contained some 5-nucleotidase. Finally the endothelium of the blood capillaries contained alkaline phosphatase but none of the above enzymes. Barka *et al.* (1961) noted the presence of acid phosphatase in lymph nodes as in other reticuloendothelial organs and put forward the view that acid phosphatase could be considered as a convenient marker of reticuloendothelial cells.

Ballantyne (1967) found a non-specific esterase (sensitive to E600 and to mipafox) in cells with elongated processes in the marginal sinuses, at the periphery of lymphoid nodules, in the diffuse cortical lymphoid tissue, and in the medulla, notably its outer part. A positive reaction for esterase was also present in blood capillaries and post capillary venules. Cholinesterase was found in rather similar sites in the cortex only. Ballantyne and Burwell (1965) speculated that these enzymes were involved in the degradation and disposal of potentially toxic esters. These they thought were produced as a result of lipid metabolism in mitosis, either in the tissues draining to the node, or in the germinal centres of the lymph node itself.

Menzies (1965) has suggested on the basis of the electron microscopic observations of others that the "skeleton of a lymph node is a protoplasmic pseudo-syncytium, made up of the interlacing membranous processes of dendritic macrophages, with fibres running in extra-cytoplasmic tunnels and providing occasional reinforcement". He claims that this framework can be demonstrated by briefly "staining" unfixed frozen sections of lymph nodes with Pelikan ink. The carbon adheres selectively to the bodies and processes of macrophages, leaving lymphoid cells almost completely unmarked". It is clear that this technique outlines the finest connective tissue framework of the node but not certain that it outlines dendritic macrophages. It is not certain or indeed likely that all of the cells whose cytoplasmic processes cover the connective tissue framework of the node are dendritic antigen-trapping macrophages in the sense of Maruyama and Masuda (1964) or Nossal *et al.* (1968a, b).

The early literature on the ultrastructure of lymph nodes has been reviewed elsewhere (Carr, 1970). There is common agreement from the work of Sorenson (1960); Clark (1962); Toro and Rohlich (1962); Moe (1963, 1964) and Mori (1966) among others that the sinusoids of a lymph node are lined partly by poorly phagocytic endothelial cells and partly by more highly phagocytic macrophages (Fig. 22). There are often gaps between the lining cells, though adjacent endothelial cells are often held together by desmosomes. Collagen fibres lie deep to the cells lining sinusoids and traverse both the extrasinusoidal parenchyma and the sinusoids. In both situations the collagen is covered by the cytoplasm of cells; some of these cells look like typical fibroblasts while elsewhere they look like typical macrophages. There is no good evidence that cells can be both avidly phagocytic (viz. macrophages) and synthesize collagen.

Macrophages are found lining sinusoids, both cortical and medullary, immediately outside the basement membrane of sinusoids and lying in a true interstitial position either in lymphoid tissue or within germinal centres. There is no very good evidence of striking differences between these cells, but sufficient detailed ultrastructural investigation has not been done.

The typical lymph node macrophage has an irregular surface with numerous flap-like ruffles (Fig. 23). The best developed of these are seen in the subcapsular sinus, where they may be circular in cross section, and derive from macrophages, either within or outside the sinus wall.

Dense bodies probably lysosomal are numerous. Most are small, demarcated by a unit membrane, and contain granular electron dense material in which ferritin is scarce or absent. At least the smallest of these as suggested by Onoe and Tsukada (1964) are probably primary lysosomes. However when tracer particles are injected into the footpad of the mouse and the popliteal lymph node is examined, particles are found in quite small homogeneous dense bodies; this suggests ready connection between these structures and micropinocytic vesicles.

The larger dense bodies are clearly secondary lysosomes, containing aggregates of ferritin, myelin figures and fragments of cellular debris. Such structures are not as numerous in lymph node macrophages as in those of spleen (Figs 24 and 25).

Several types of vesicular structure are present; the largest lie near the surface and are indentations or vesicles nearly 1 μm in diameter. These may represent true pinocytosis. Smaller vesicles 60–100 nm are frequent, both near the surface and deeper in the cell. In addition there are a few bristle coated vesicles 100–180 nm in diameter and usually near the cell surface. The granular endoplasmic reticulum and Golgi apparatus are usually fairly prominent, and mitochondria are of the normal elongated pattern.

A prominent feature of many lymph node macrophages is a well developed microfibrillar apparatus. The fibrils measure 4–6 nm in diameter, a size consistent with the view that these are actin filaments; they are homogeneous in structure without periodicity; they run in bundles, joining and branching. The surface ectoplasm, notably the flaps which lie in the subcapsular sinus, shows a network of microfibrils which in places run at right angles to the cell membrane and lie very close to it. While there is no unequivocal evidence of actual attachment it seems very likely that there is some form of attachment between microfibril and membrane (Fig. 26).

These cells also contain complex aggregates of microtubules some 25 nm in diameter again lying in bundles with some evidence of branching. Microfibrils are found in close relationship to these microtubular aggregates. The function of these structures is not certain but it seems reasonable to suppose that the fibrils represent contractile elements and that the tubules may be cytoskeletal (Fig. 27) (Carr, 1972).

Apart from ordinary macrophages a group of cells has been described in lymph nodes as dendritic reticular cells or better dendritic macrophages. These are quite distinct from ordinary macrophages.

The bodies of these cells lie at the centre of the follicle. They are deeply invaginated and give off many processes which interdigitate with one another and with lymphocyte processes to form a labyrinth. Adjacent dendritic cells may be held to one another by desmosomes (Milanesi, 1965a, b; Schulze, 1965; Nossal et al., 1968b). The cytoplasm of dendritic cells commonly contains few differentiated membranous structures and few lysosomes, but considerable numbers of free ribonucleoprotein particles. The web of dendritic processes may arise from cells at different levels of differentiation; according to Mori et al. (1969, 1971) dendritic cells may be either truly primitive undifferentiated mesenchymal cells, "reticulum cells" in his terminology, or very immature cells committed along the lymphocyte line of differentiation. This distinction is doubtful, but it seems at present unwise to be dogmatic as to whether dendritic cells really are macrophages. These cells, as discussed later, bind antigen in sensitized animals.

Within lymphoid follicles in addition to dendritic cells variable numbers of ordinary macrophages are found, containing large inclusions which can be seen at the ultrastructural level to be composed of degenerating cells, mostly lymphocytes, in various stages of degradation. These so called "tingible" bodies are best seen in lymph nodes undergoing immunological reactions, where the cell turnover is high.

The effects of irradiation of a lymph node have been studied by Smith *et al.* (1967). The macrophages developed numerous prominent pseudopodia, presumably in reaction to the more radiosensitive lymphocytes degenerating around them.

Microglia

The existence of mesodermal connective tissue elements scattered among the neuroectoderm of the central nervous system was hinted at by various nineteenth and early twentieth century authors notably Robertson (1900) but the widespread recognition of a phagocytic and mesodermal element is the result of the work of Hortega in the years 1919–1921 summarized in his extensive review (1932). This review and Glees' monograph (1955) may be consulted for the early literature on the topic. Hortega showed that there was a widespread element in the mammalian central nervous system which stained specifically by a silver carbonate technique and further that in the main these cells could be recognized in conventional microscopic preparations by their densely staining polymorphous nuclei. He studied these cells in embryonic and adult animals and in various pathological conditions and showed that they could be regarded as a discrete functional entity.

Microglial cells are found scattered throughout the nervous system as single cells, usually multipolar, with three to six processes which arborize and whose branches are covered with numerous thin twigs. Bipolar, unipolar, and flattened lamellar variants are sometimes found, and there are minor variations in size and structure in different parts of the nervous system; more microglial cells are present in some parts of the central nervous system than in others.

The microglial cells migrate into the nervous system from the meninges in late foetal life, in the main at fairly restricted sites: the tela chorioidea (of all the ventricles) and the pia over the cerebral peduncles. Hortega was unable to identify with certainty the nature of these "microglioblasts" but described them as "morphologically similar to lymphocytes" and as "polyblastic cells capable of migration through amoeboid movements and formation of pseudopodia which after some time became macrophages". This view is still acceptable in the light of modern ideas on the genesis of macrophages elsewhere. Later work on the affinity for silver stains of the reticulo-endothelial elements would suggest that contact with nervous tissue (as suggested by Hortega, 1932) is not necessary for the development of this affinity for silver stains. Round or amoeboid microglial elements are present for some time in the young animal, presumably immature forms. The mesodermal origin of microglia has been confirmed by several workers, notably Dougherty (1944).

In various pathological reactions Hortega described the presence of enlarged microglial elements. The cells enlarge, their processes become shorter and shorter, and finally they become roughly ovoid with typical pseudopodia and contain phagocytosed material of various types, iron and fat globules. Hortega regarded these elements in various acute lesions as microglia; clearly many of them are, but it is of course impossible to distinguish which are haematogenous elements. Since however, it is likely that microglia ultimately come from the blood stream this is not of great importance. A microglial cell is a macrophage and like any macrophage in any lesion, a microglial cell in an inflammatory focus in the brain may have left the circulation either recently or in the distant past. It is not known how long microglia live or whether they divide. In chronic nervous lesions of various types the microglia may increase greatly in numbers and become elongated and rod-like ("*stabchenzellen*") possibly because they have pulled in their processes and are squeezing through narrow spaces (Hortega, 1932).

Field (1957) studied small puncture wounds in the cerebrum and showed that leucocytic infiltration was minimal; he suggested that compound granular corpuscles, the macrophages of brain lesions, might derive from either microglia or oligodendroglia. Konigsmark and Sidman (1963) in a similar experiment used labelling with tritiated thymidine to disprove this view and show conclusively that compound granular corpuscles were haematogenous.

It is clear that microglia can phagocytose red blood cells or cellular debris. Hortega (1932) suggested that the microglia could be regarded as part of the reticulo-endothelial system. He pointed out that at that date the evidence as to whether microglia could clear colloids from the blood stream was conflicting; before microglial cells can phagocytose circulating colloids, the colloids must be able to escape from the circulation, e.g. in the region of a wound where, as is now known, the blood vessels leak (Russell, 1929). Jaffe (1938) however did not admit that microglial cells were part of the RES.

The identity of the microglia with macrophages was strongly supported by the work of Wells and Carmichael (1930). These workers cultured the brains of fowl embryos and studied the cells by vital staining and silver impregnation. Cells grew in culture very similar indeed to microglia and showing a selective affinity for vital dyes and silver stains. Wolfgram and Rose (1957) came to rather similar conclusions. Russell (1929) showed that after making a sterile puncture wound of the rabbit brain many cells appeared round the wound showing all stages of transition in appearance between microglia and mature fat-laden macrophages. These cells had a marked affinity for trypan blue. Penfield (1925) showed that microglia in gliomas were actively phagocytic.

In addition to microglia Kubie (1927) showed by neutral red supravital staining that lymphocytes and clasmatocytes lay immediately round the blood vessels in the guinea-pig brain.

The earlier electron micrographs of microglia (Luse, 1956; Schulz et al., 1957; Herndon, 1964) show a small undifferentiated cell often irregular in shape. The nucleus may be notably dense (Farquar and Hartmann, 1957). More mature macrophages exist in brain only in relation to some pathological lesion. They then resemble macrophages elsewhere, but often contain considerable residues of undigested myelin. It is of course not then possible to distinguish those of microglial origin from those of monocytic origin (Gonatas et al., 1963, 1964; Blinzinger and Kreutzberg, 1968).

Mori and Leblond (1969) examined the microglia in the corpus callosum of the rat with the electron microscope after carrying out the classical silver staining technique. The cells identified by silver staining as microglia had a small nucleus with densely staining chromatin and considerable numbers of dense bodies, presumably lysosomes. Some microglia are found within the basement membrane of capillaries; these (pericytic) microglia have little cytoplasm, few dense bodies and few processes; others lie scattered singly within the brain tissue proper, sending off long processes between adjacent cells. The latter (interstitial) microglia contain numerous dense bodies and may derive from the pericytic cells. These cells did not take up tritiated thymidine (Figs 31 and 32).

In addition to microglia actually within the brain substance, a considerable number of macrophages lie in the connective tissue of the choroidal plexuses (Jayatilaka, 1965). These cells have prominent cytoplasmic processes and bear a considerable resemblance to Hofbauer cells (see below) (Fig. 30).

Placental Macrophages

The presence of vacuolated elliptical cells in the mesodermal core of the placental villi has been known since the latter years of the nineteenth century. These cells were thought by Hofbauer (1925) to be a type of histiocyte. Lewis (1924) showed very clearly that when human placental villi were cut into fragments and incubated in neutral red, these cells concentrated the dye notably. Their ultrastructure was described in detail by Wynn (1967), Luckett (1970) and Enders and King (1970). The latter authors give good brief reviews of the literature to date.

Hofbauer cells are found in the largest numbers in immature placentas (from the sixth to twentieth week in the human) (Lewis, 1924) but are present (Fox, 1967) in the villi of more than 80% of normal placentas at term, in over 90% of placentas from premature deliveries and in 100% of placentas from diabetic mothers or mothers with Rh incompatibility.

They are plump ovoid eosinophilic cells which like macrophages elsewhere contain large quantities of acid phosphatase. Their general ultrastructure is that of macrophages (Fig. 33) but they have unusually large cytoplasmic flanges, large vacuoles, and numerous micropinocytotic vesicles. When horseradish peroxidase is injected into the maternal circulation it is found in the micropinocytotic vesicles and vacuoles of Hofbauer cells. Hofbauer cells can be obtained from tissue cultures of the placenta (Fox and Kharkongor, 1970) (Fig. 30).

The function of these placental macrophages is uncertain. It is obviously possible that they may be involved in the removal of bacteria from the placenta. Enders and King (1970) point out that the placental disc lacks lymphatics and suggests that they may sequester foetal serum proteins in the stroma of the chorionic villus. Another function that has been demonstrated is the phagocytosis of meconium; the significance of this is not clear.

Metalophilia

Many macrophages at numerous sites have an affinity for silver stains—so called metalophilic macrophages. This phenomenon will be discussed here for convenience; some of this information is duplicated in other sections. Early investigations on this were carried out by Hortega and an extensive investigation was made by Dunning and Stevenson (1934). Small metalophilic cells were present in normal liver spleen and kidney. After injury to these organs metalophilic cells were prominent in the inflammatory reaction. Some of these were small; other clearly larger forms showed evidence of phagocytosis. Dunning and Furth (1935) examined cultures of monocytes and peritoneal cells by the same techniques and showed transitional forms which suggested transitions from monocytes to macrophages. Similar cells were demonstrated in the pulmonary alveolar walls by Gazayerli (1936). Marshall (1946) re-examined the pulmonary metalophil cells in greater detail and showed that there were two types—branched cells found in the paravascular and peribronchial tissues and rounded cells found both in the interstitial tissues and in the alveolar lumen.

Marshall (1956) later studied the whole of the reticulo-endothelial system by the silver impregnation technique. He found that the metalophil cells in the tissue could be divided into fixed and amoeboid. In addition a few (but only a few) of the blood monocytes stained positively. Fixed metalophils were of two types—solitary and syncytial. The solitary cells included the CNS microglia, the Kupffer cells, and cells in the omentum, marrow, lung, thymic medulla, and the spleen—mainly in the white pulp, but to a lesser extent in the red pulp. These cells had an oval or rod-shaped nucleus; their cytoplasm was elongated with lateral branches of variable extent. They often lay round blood vessels. In the sinuses of the lymph nodes and the spleen the metalophil cells appeared to be syncytial, though recent work with the electron miscoscope has not confirmed this. The "amoeboid" cells had a round nucleus with round or oval cytoplasm.

In the spleen (Marshall and White, 1950) metalophil cells were very numerous, notably in the red pulp where amoeboid cells, branching cells and sinus lining cells could be distinguished. In addition fine branching cells were present at the periphery of the white pulp. In lymph nodes sinus lining cells and solitary medullary metalophils could be distinguished, and similarly in the bone marrow some of the metalophil cells clearly lined sinusoids. In inflammatory lesions both mononuclear cells and branching histiocytes were metalophilic. When animals which had received a dose of a vital dye were studied the metalophilic cells were often but not always those which had taken up the vital dyes. There were more metalophils than cells which took up colloids. Polymorphs notably do not stain by the silver carbonate technique. Marshall considered that metalophilia was a fundamental property of a group of cells, perhaps more fundamental than colloid uptake. "The reticulo-endothelial system is not a distinct cytological entity, but a functional state of some metalophil cells, due either to properties of the cells themselves, or to the nature of the local blood and lymph circulation."

The metalophils are very well demonstrated in the spleen, for instance at the junction of white and red pulp, the marginal metalophils of Snook (1964). These cells are not avidly phagocytic. Acid phosphatase and non-specific esterase is present in and characteristic of reticuloendothelial cells (Gomori, 1941; Barka et al., 1961). Pettersen (1964) compared the distribution of cells containing these enzymes in the rat spleen with the distribution of metalophil cells. In a study of spleens from normal animals and from animals treated with TAB vaccine and other stimulants, he found that the marginal metalophilic cells had a positive acid phosphatase reaction, but only a weakly positive esterase reaction. In the lymphoid nodules rather more than a half of the metalophilic cells gave a positive acid phosphatase reaction and less than a quarter gave a positive esterase reaction. Stimulation produced an increase in the number of cells giving a positive histochemical reaction for the enzymes but not an increase in the number of metalophilic cells. The changes on stimulation were much more prominent in the white pulp than in the red pulp.

The development of the metalophilic cells of rat spleen has been studied by McFadden (1968). No metalophilic cells and no cells containing histochemically demonstrable acid phosphatase or esterase were present in the foetal spleen. During early postnatal growth metalophilic cells became evident before cells containing acid hydrolytic enzymes. Very primitive macrophage precursors are probably not metalophilic (Marshall, 1956).

From these findings it seems reasonable to regard metalophilia as a property of some macrophages which develops during maturation, at a stage before the appearance of a sufficient quantity of acid hydrolytic enzymes—i.e. lysosomes—to be histochemically demonstrable. The things which make a cell stain with silver carbonate are not known. It is unlikely that the reaction is very highly specific. The cell coats of many cells stain with silver stains (Rambourg and Leblond, 1965) and macrophages certainly have prominent cell coats (Carr et al., 1970). Also lysosomes and other secretion granules often stain well with silver stains. Which, if either, of these properties is related to the metalophilia of Hortega and Marshall, a much grosser phenomenon, is not certain. The only EM study of metalophilia carried out on microglial cells by Mori and Leblond (1969) showed that the silver was deposited in rather large non-specific precipitates.

In summary, "fixed" macrophages are found in the main in the lymphoreticular organs of the body—the spleen, the lymph nodes, the marrow and the liver. There is a general overall similarity in their structure and behaviour; they are actively phagocytic and therefore contain ingested material and therefore also require hydrolytic enzymes for the digestion of this material. They possess the cytoplasmic apparatus for the synthesis of these enzymes and are often metalophilic.

A major function is to monitor streams of fluid which flow past them; they may either line a blood vessel as in the liver, or be found adjacent to a blood vessel which frequently leaks as in the spleen. In the lymph node they are found both lining the lymphatic sinusoids or outside them. Finally though "fixed" during their normal functions, there is ample evidence that at least some of them may arise elsewhere probably in the marrow, circulate and settle out in the peripheral lympho-reticular organs and further that they may very occasionally regain their freedom and recirculate at least to the lungs. The physiological significance of the latter is not certain.

An interesting subgroup of cells which can almost certainly be regarded as a variant of the histiocyte are the cells of Langerhans (Breathnach *et al.*, 1964 reviewed by Breathnach, 1965) (Fig. 34). These are found in the epidermis and were initially identified by their affinity for heavy metal salts. They contain characteristic rod-shaped inclusions 160–1600 nm long by 30–50 nm wide (in a given section) bounded by membrane and containing a central electron dense core in which a periodicity of about 9 nm can sometimes be made out; the interior of the inclusion can sometimes be shown to be continuous with extracellular space, suggesting that this may be a complex micropinocytotic phenomenon. Reconstructions from serial sections have suggested that these inclusions are in fact disc shaped or cup shaped and that the core is paracrystalline (Wolff, 1967; Sagebiel and Reed, 1968). Similar cells have been observed in a group of uncommon human disorders, the histiocytoses (see Chapter Fourteen).

Chapter Three

THE ORIGIN AND CIRCULATION
OF THE MACROPHAGE

Since Metchnikoff's day numerous workers have investigated and speculated as to whether macrophages arise locally from connective tissue or
endothelial cell precursors (Aschoff, 1924; Foot, 1925) or from a circulating precursor whether a lymphocyte, a monocyte or a small mononuclear
cell which could not be defined as truly lymphocytic or monocytic, the
polyblast (Maximow, 1928) (see Roser, 1970; van Furth, 1970 for reviews).

A good morphological study representative of the earlier work was that
of Kolouth (1939); in the first few hours after subcutaneous injection of
albumen large macrophages were present which could only have arisen
locally; later transitional cells between lymphocyte and macrophage were
seen.

Evidence of lymphocyte–macrophage transformation has come from
tissue culture studies. Bloom (1938) found such transformations in
thoracic duct lymphocytes cultured *in vitro;* but his results were ascribed
by Medawar (1940) to contamination by tissue cells during collection of
the cells from the thoracic duct. When human peripheral leucocytes are
cultured *in vitro* a series of morphological intermediates occurs between
small lymphocytes and actively phagocytic cells, which are however
morphologically different from macrophages as seen in the intact animal
(Chapman *et al.*, 1967a, b).

Rebuck *et al.* (1955, 1960) studied the cells which migrated on to glass
coverslips covering small experimental abrasions of the skin surface. The
lesion could be challenged with such substances as typhoid vaccine, diphtheria toxoid or tuberculin and the phagocytic powers of the cells in the
exudate tested with vital dyes such as trypan blue or lithium carmine.

The exudate initially was composed largely of neutrophilic polymorphs,
followed by lymphocytes and some monocytes. As time passed more large

41

lymphocytes gathered and these were seen to store dyes; ultimately the
lesions contained numerous dye-storing macrophages. Transitional forms
between large dye-storing lymphocytes and macrophages were found. The
illustrations in Rebuck's papers are extremely convincing and, providing
it be remembered that at no point does he prove (or even claim) either
that all blood lymphocytes can mature into macrophages, or that all macrophages derive from lymphocytes, then his main conclusions must be
accepted.

The proportion of lymphocytes which can turn into macrophages is
important. Holub (1962) studied rabbit thoracic duct lymphocytes in a
diffusion chamber and found that less than 10% of them could change into
macrophages both morphologically and functionally, when autotrans-
planted; and that a similar proportion could change into plasma cells when
homotransplanted with or without protein antigen.

The crux of the argument as to whether lymphocytes can turn into
macrophages probably lies in definition. Maximow (1928) used the term
polyblast to denote the small precursor of a macrophage whether lymphoid
or monocytic. It is true that some cells which look in the light microscope
like lymphocytes can turn into macrophages; these lymphocytes if examined with the electron microscope would probably show the ultrastructure of monocytes.

The migration of monocytes from the circulation in the rabbit ear
chamber, and their maturation into macrophages, has been clearly
demonstrated by phase contrast microscopy of living tissue (Ebert and
Florey, 1939) and by electron microscopy (Cliff, 1963).

The Monocyte

It is currently held that the most important precursor of the macrophage
is the circulating blood monocyte; but before examining this proposition
in detail, it is as well to arrive at some definition of the monocyte. It is a
rather poorly phagocytic cell some 12 μm (10–20 μm) in diameter with an
indented nucleus and small azurophil inclusions. When stained intravitally
with neutral red, there is a small central rosette of granules; it gives a
positive reaction to the periodic acid Schiff technique, probably largely
due to the glycoprotein in its lysosomes and a positive peroxidase reaction
(Brucher, 1958). It is difficult to identify monocytes absolutely in a tissue
section.

The ultrastructure of monocytes has been described by several authors; (Low and Freeman, 1958; Bessis and Thiery, 1961; Wiener *et al.*, 1965; Zucker-Franklin *et al.*, 1966; Watanabe *et al.*, 1967; van Furth *et al.*, 1970; Nichols *et al.*, 1971). The monocyte has a relatively smooth surface with a few small finger-like cytoplasmic processes. Several oval or round mitochondria are visible in a section. Granular endoplasmic reticulum is present in small amounts; the Golgi apparatus is composed of rows of flattened sacs. Small vesicles are scattered throughout the cell and the surface may show indentations, presenting as apparent vacuoles. All of these membranous elements are much less prominent than in macrophages, but more prominent than in lymphocytes. Polyribosomes are relatively few in the circulating monocyte. Accounts of the number of membrane bound dense bodies vary from species to species. Most monocytes show at least one or two lysosomal dense bodies in a single section of the cell (Fig. 36).

The existence of a rapidly dividing monocyte precursor in the bone marrow has recently been demonstrated (van Furth and Cohn, 1968; van Furth *et al.*, 1970; van Furth and Dulk, 1970). These cells label rapidly with thymidine and are slightly larger than monocytes; they have numerous polyribosomes and a prominent Golgi apparatus but little granular endoplasmic reticulum.

Nichols *et al.* (1971) have studied in detail the differentiation of monocytes, in the rabbit, the guinea-pig and man. The promonocyte found in the marrow is slightly larger (7–15 μm) than the mature cell. As would be expected in an immature cell it has a large nucleus with several nucleolar profiles; the cytoplasm has numerous free polysomes and a conspicuous Golgi complex but little rough endoplasmic reticulum. Many small round or ovoid electron-dense membrane-bound granules 100–500 nm are found in these cells; these are the azurophil granules of the light microscopist. Some of the Golgi vesicles have a finely granular electron-dense content similar to that of the granules. This is presumptive evidence that the azurophil granules are secretory granules whose contents are concentrated in the Golgi complex as happens in other secretory systems. The more mature circulating monocyte is smaller (9–11 μm) with a relatively smaller nucleus and fewer free polysomes. Azurophil dense granules may be more numerous, and a little denser; their average size is a little larger. The endoplasmic reticulum, the Golgi zone and sometimes the perinuclear zone of these cells gave a positive reaction for acid phosphatase and aryl sulphatase and positive reactions for both of these enzymes were found in the immature granules. The mature granules on the other hand gave a posi-tive reaction for aryl sulphatase. Peroxidase was found in similar situations. In both cases there were considerable species differences. Peritoneal exudate macrophages from rabbits and guinea-pigs similarly show prominent re-actions for these enzymes but do not however show azurophil granules; appearances were seen which suggested that small coated vesicles acted as primary lysosomes to carry hydrolytic enzymes from the Golgi complex to secondary lysosomes. Nichols *et al.* (1971) have therefore suggested that cells of the monocyte–macrophage series produce two distinct types of primary lysosome, during different phases of its life cycle—azurophil granules in bone marrow or blood, and coated vesicles in tissues and body cavities. There is good evidence however (Carr, 1968a, b) that azurophil granules similar to those in monocytes exist in considerable numbers in peritoneal and other macrophages. Hirsch and Fedorko (1970) suggest that peroxidase staining granules are numerous in the promonocyte, fewer in the monocyte and absent in the more mature macrophages.

Monocytes have been isolated in quantity from the blood by centri-fugation in concentrated albumen solutions. With the appropriate con-centration of albumin a pellet of monocytes and lymphocytes is obtained. The cells are allowed to settle on a glass surface. When they are washed it is alleged that only the monocytes stick to the surface. It should be noted however that there is no absolute proof that some cells which on morpho-logic criteria should be called lymphocytes do not stick to glass (Bennett and Cohn, 1966; Cline and Lehrer, 1968). When monocytes are cultured *in vitro* there is an increase in cell size and in the number of mitochondria, an increase in content of cytochrome oxidase, acid phosphatase and aryl sulphatase and in utilization of glucose and production of lactic acid. As the cells mature *in vitro* they become more actively phagocytic.

If the circulating monocyte is the precursor of the tissue macrophage it is of some interest to know how long it normally lives in the circulation when there is no significant inflammatory lesion present to draw off mono-cytes in large numbers. This has been studied in the rat (Whitelaw, 1966) and in the mouse (van Furth and Cohn, 1968; van Furth and Dulk, 1970; van Furth, 1970) by labelling with tritiated thymidine. The half-life of a monocyte in the circulation has been reckoned at 72 h in the mouse and 12 h in the rat. The disappearance of labelled cells from the circulation occurred in accordance with an exponential function, suggesting that they were transformed or left the circulation at random.

The Origin of Macrophages in Inflammation

The origin of macrophages in inflammatory lesions has been extensively studied by administering tritiated thymidine to animals and making auto-radiographs of inflammatory lesions. Thus in inflammatory reactions induced by injecting various proteins into skin there were many labelled cells present; the cells engaged in DNA synthesis may so far as can be seen by light microscopy be large lymphocytes or monocytes. When delayed hypersensitivity is transferred from one animal to another by means of cells, most of the cells in hypersensitive inflammatory lesions in the host animal were recently proliferated cells of host origin (Goldman and Walker, 1963; Kosunen *et al.*, 1963a). Further evidence on the haematogenous origin of macrophages was obtained by implanting glass coverslips in the subcutaneous tissues of rats; when tritiated thymidine was given 18–21 h before the coverslip was removed some 60% of the macrophages on the coverslip were labelled. Irradiation of the marrow grossly reduced the number of labelled macrophages present; this deficiency was restored by the infusion of cells from marrow or spleen. Removal of the lymphoreticular organs did not affect cellular exudates on coverslips (Volkman and Gowans, 1965a, b). It was clear from these experiments that most of the precursors of macrophages were monocytes, but possible that some might have been small lymphocytes. By similar techniques Volkman (1966) demonstrated the marrow origin of many of the mononuclear cells in rat peritoneal exudates. Similarly in the inflammatory lesion induced by subcutaneous injection of fibrinogen, most of the macrophages derived from blood monocytes; most of the latter came from precursors which had recently divided. Probably polymorphs and monocytes migrate randomly; the former die or migrate away; the latter persist, enlarge and mature into macrophages (Paz and Spector, 1962; Spector *et al.*, 1965). Macrophages in the mouse similarly were shown by labelling techniques to derive from a rapidly dividing marrow precursor (van Furth and Cohn, 1968).

Since macrophages in inflammation derive from monocytes, clearly they will be affected by anything which affects the blood monocyte count. Thus the number of circulating monocytes is reduced by treatment with glucocorticoids (Thompson and van Furth, 1970).

There is conflicting evidence on the mitotic potential of mature macrophages. Thus van Furth and Cohn (1968) suggested that peripheral blood monocytes and peritoneal macrophages in the mouse were end cells and did not divide. On the other hand Forbes and Mackaness (1963) demon-strated mitosis in peritoneal macrophages and Khoo and Mackaness (1964) showed marked proliferation in peritoneal cells after systemic intravenous infection with *Listeria* and *Brucella*. Here there was no induction of a local peritoneal inflammatory response. Wiener (1967) has correlated DNA synthesis in peritoneal cells with cellular acid phosphatase activity. DNA synthesis was found only in morphologically well differentiated macro-phages. Aronson and Elberg (1962) after injecting oil into the peritoneum showed that a high percentage of labelled histiocytes (i.e. large macro-phages) were present. They interpreted these findings to mean local formation of histiocytes. While other interpretations are possible, the hypothesis that a significant number of peritoneal macrophages may ori-ginate locally, possibly from the milk spots, is supported by the demon-stration (Aronson and Shahar, 1965) that macrophages are formed in considerable numbers in the isolated omentum *in vitro*.

The availability of closely inbred strains of laboratory animals permitted another approach to the problem of the origin of macrophages. With such inbred strains it is possible to raise an antiserum which will specifically kill the cells of one strain of mouse but not of another. When animals of one strain are irradiated to kill their haemopoietic cells, and these cells replaced by haemopoietic cells of another strain, then in the resulting chimera it becomes possible to identify cells originating from one or the other strain by use of the appropriate antiserum.

Thus Goodman (1964) gave mice a single lethal dose of whole body radiation and after 24 h injected haemopoietic cells from one of several sources: bone marrow, white blood cells, foetal liver cells and peritoneal fluid cells. Three months or more after grafting, peritoneal cells were all killed by anti-donor serum but not by anti-host serum. In a similar set of experiments Balner (1963) noted that only the macrophages, not the lymphocytes in the peritoneal fluid survived the initial irradiation. For the first 10 days after irradiation nearly all the peritoneal cells were of host type but thereafter they were gradually replaced by donor cells till at 6 weeks only donor cells were present.

Virolainen (1968) has studied mouse radiation chimeras, by the marker chromosome technique. The strain of mice from which the donor cells were derived carries a marker chromosome readily identifiable in dividing cells in tissue culture. The conclusion was reached that macrophages through-out the body are derived from bone marrow. The inherent disadvantage of the technique is of course that only dividing cells are identified; the conclusion is indisputable but of course does not necessarily mean that *all* macrophages derive immediately from marrow.

The Origin of Kupffer Cells

The origin of Kupffer cells has been a matter of debate for many years. Under normal circumstances some 0·7% of Kupffer cells take up tritiated thymidine (Shorter and Titus, 1962); there is marked proliferation after stimulation for instance with glucan (Ashworth *et al.*, 1963). As early as 1927 de Haan and Hoekstra showed that macrophages labelled with particles would settle out in the walls of hepatic sinusoids. Roser (1965) using macrophages labelled with radioactive colloids confirmed this view.

This is not however the same as proving that Kupffer cells normally do arise from a distant precursor. Howard and his group have studied the origin of Kupffer cells by isolating them from the liver by enzymatic digestion, culturing them and examining their chromosomal constitution. When under a variety of extreme and sometimes rather artificial forms of reticuloendothelial stimulation, animals were given marrow or thoracic duct cells labelled with the readily identifiable T6 marker chromosome, it was clearly shown that Kupffer cells could derive from precursors in thoracic duct lymph or bone marrow (Howard, 1963; Boak *et al.*, 1968; Kinsky *et al.*, 1969).

On the other hand the proliferation of Kupffer cells induced by oestrogen stimulation is inhibited by local irradiation of the liver, strongly suggesting local replication of Kupffer cells (Kelly *et al.*, 1962; Kelly and Dobson, 1971). Similarly during the development of immunity to *Listeria*, Kupffer cells can divide locally (North, 1969b).

The general conclusion must be that under stimulation Kupffer cells may originate immediately from marrow precursors; under extreme stimulation, they may derive from recirculating cells in lymph. It seems likely however that local division of Kupffer cells is an important, if not the most important mechanism of day to day replacement.

The Origin of Pulmonary Macrophages

The origin of the pulmonary macrophages has aroused much controversy; early work is reviewed by Bertalanaffy (1964a, b). Possible sources include alveolar epithelial cells, interstitial connective tissue cells in the lung parenchyma, vascular endothelial cells and blood monocytes. Gazayerli (1936) and Marshall (1946) studied the pulmonary phagocytes by silver impregnation techniques. The former author showed that septal cells stained with silver; the latter traced a sequence of development between local mesenchymal precursors and phagocytes. Marshall concluded that phagocytes probably were not of epithelial origin, but might derive from monocytes in inflammatory states; Bertalanaffy (1964a, b) in an exhaustive study concluded that alveolar phagocytes derived either by division from previous alveolar cells, or from mesenchymal "fibroblast-like forms in the alveolar wall".

The first attempt to determine the origin of lung macrophages experimentally was that of Ungar and Wilson (1935). These workers marked guinea-pig peritoneal exudate mononuclear cells by labelling with lithium carmine, and then injected them into the heart of another guinea-pig. More than 50% of the cells were viable after carmine labelling as determined by further labelling with carbon. Most of the carmine labelled cells were found to settle in the lungs, some in the stroma, some in the alveolar walls but most in the alveolar spaces. This experiment suggests that under normal circumstances alveolar phagocytes might derive from some source similar to peritoneal macrophages; the experiment however is a rather unnatural one.

More recently Shorter et al. (1966) have studied cell turnover in the pulmonary alveolus after administration of tritiated thymidine and have established that there are two distinct populations of cells. The turnover time of alveolar epithelial cells is about 7 days while that of true macrophages is much longer, about 35 days.

The origin of lung macrophages has been further studied by Pinkett et al. (1966) using chromosome marker techniques. CBA mice were irradiated and given injections of bone marrow cells carrying the T6 marker chromosome. After 1–4 months about two thirds of the alveolar macrophages were clearly of host origin. This establishes unequivocally that many lung macrophages are ultimately of marrow origin. However there is not an immediate depletion of lung macrophages after marrow irradiation and it seems that while lung macrophages derive ultimately from marrow they are held for a considerable time in the interstitial tissue of the lung and indeed divide there (Bowden et al., 1969).

The Origin of Brain Macrophages

Large macrophages, "*gitterzellen*" or compound granular corpuscles appear in the brain in various pathological circumstances (see review by Russell,

1962). The classical view is that these derive largely from the microglia. This problem has been re-investigated by Konigsmark and Sidman (1966). After repeated doses of tritiated thymidine few labelled cells were found in the normal brain. After a stab wound had been made in the brain large numbers of labelled macrophages appeared in the wound. Correlation of the sequential changes in the percentage of labelled macrophages in the wound and the percentage of circulating labelled leucocytes indicated that about two thirds of the macrophages were derived from circulating mononuclear leucocytes. A few might have derived from circulating lymphocytes but most of the rest probably originated from local microglia. Similarly Adrian and Walker (1962) showed that macrophages in injured spinal cord were labelled after injection of tritiated thymidine. Kosunen et al. (1963b) studied experimental allergic encephalomyelitis in the rat. A large proportion of the cells of the perivascular infiltrate were labelled by injection of tritiated thymidine one or more days before lesion formation begins. These cells were medium or large blood lymphocytes which developed into histiocytes as the lesion was evolving. Russell (1962) used the electron microscope to study the cells which appeared in a cortical stab wound; a series of appearances was traced from a typical blood monocyte to the typical brain macrophage or *"gitter"* cell.

Circulation of Mature Macrophages

Mature macrophages can circulate, but the importance of this is doubtful. A few mature macrophages may be found in the circulation in the normal animal, even the normal human. These are very large cells 15–30 μm in diameter, with a notably kidney-shaped nucleus and containing lipid and phagocytosed material (Jaffe, 1938; Herbeuval Bolikowska et al., 1966).

After repeated intravenous injection of colloids into rats, showers of macrophages appear in the circulating blood, probably arising from liver and spleen (Simpson, 1922). Under similar circumstances Kupffer cells may migrate to the lungs (Irwin, 1932).

When peritoneal macrophages were labelled with a colloid and injected intravenously they were found to settle largely in the hepatic sinusoids (de Haan and Hoekstra, 1927). Nicol and Bilbey (1958) pretreated mice with repeated doses of oestradiol and then gave them carbon intravenously. Carbon-laden macrophages were found thereafter in blood from the right side of the heart but not from the left side of the heart. Sequential examination of animals showed early localization to liver and spleen, followed later by the appearance of large numbers of carbon-bearing macrophages in the lungs and the passage of carbon-bearing cells into the alveoli. Both carbon-bearing cells and carbon were recovered from bronchial washings. Schneeberger-Keeley and Burger (1970) provided very strong evidence of circulation of Kupffer cells. These authors found numerous phagocytic cells exhibiting micropinocytosis vermiformis in the pulmonary capillaries of cats with experimental pulmonary oedema, subjected to open chest ventilation. If a week before inducing the pulmonary oedema the animals had had their Kupffer cells labelled by the injection of a carbon suspension into the portal vein, numerous carbon-laden cells exhibiting micropinocytosis vermiformis were found in the lungs. This seems to prove beyond doubt that Kupffer cells can migrate. There are probably considerable species differences in the readiness with which these macrophage migrations occur. The clearance of pulmonary alveolar macrophages has been measured by Spritzer *et al.* (1964, 1968) by cannulating the oesophagus and counting the macrophages obtained; the figure arrived at was between 1 million and 3 million per hour. Roser (1965) has studied the behaviour of labelled macrophages when injected into syngeneic recipients. Peritoneal macrophages were labelled *in vivo* with radioactive colloidal gold and injected intravenously. Cell viability was checked by the ability to exclude eosin. Their distribution was established by quantitating organ radioactivity with a scintillometer, and by autoradiography. There was a brief initial period of pulmonary sequestration, after which the cells localized specifically and exclusively in liver and spleen. In relation to organ weight five times as many macrophages settled out in the spleen as settled in the liver. In the liver many of the cells had the appearance of Kupffer cells, while in the spleen they were found only in the red pulp. In the lungs they were found in the blood vessels and in the alveolar walls but not in the lumen. Heat-killed macrophages were held up longer in the lungs and the increase of radioactivity in the liver and spleen was delayed and decreased.

Alveolar macrophages were obtained by washing out the lungs and were similarly investigated (Russell and Roser, 1966). After injection they were similarly distributed but had less tendency to settle out in the spleen, and no tendency at all to settle permanently in the lungs. Kupffer cells were labelled similarly with radioactive gold and separated from the rest of the liver tissue by digestion with pronase and desoxyribonuclease followed by flotation in plasma albumen. Over 72 h more than 80% of the cells became localized in the liver of the host animal as compared with 60% of peritoneal and alveolar cells (Roser, 1968). Less than 5% of injected

Kupffer cells settled in the liver as compared with some 18% of injected peritoneal cells. It seems therefore that there is some evidence that macrophages which normally reside in a particular organ recognize and prefer the environment of that organ.

Roser (1970) has investigated the fate of peritoneal macrophage populations by injection of peritoneal macrophages labelled with radioactive gold into the peritoneal cavity. Labelled cells are found on the peritoneal milk spots within 6 h and remain there for several weeks. Labelled cells are found 12–24 h after injection in the parathymic lymph nodes, the nodes which drain the peritoneal cavity of the mouse and after a few days within the spleen. Similarly Vernon-Roberts (1969a) has shown that when carbon-labelled macrophages were injected intraperitoneally, they appeared soon thereafter in inflammatory exudates. It seems certain therefore that at least some peritoneal macrophages do not perish in the peritoneum but circulate elsewhere.

These studies establish without doubt that mature macrophages *can* circulate and also that despite any "preference" for their own organ that they can settle in another organ. They therefore contribute in a significant way to the establishment of the idea that the macrophages can be regarded as a group more united by similarities than separated by differences. The physiological importance of the circulation of mature macrophages is still not established.

Marked recirculation of macrophages may occur when the reticulo-endothelial system is stimulated—for instance in malaria (McCallum, 1969a, b). After infection with the malaria parasite, the Kupffer cells enlarge and are then shed into the circulation. They pass to the lungs where they settle out in the vascular bed, piling up on one another in the vein walls. They may then pass into the systemic circulation; little evidence was found of significant elimination by the lungs. The red cell lysis which occurs after sporulation of the parasite leads to an increase in the number of liver macrophages, partly by local differentiation, partly as a result of influx from the spleen.

The general conclusion may be reached that there is a fairly rapidly dividing stem cell in the marrow from which arises a macrophage precursor that circulates in the blood and passes into the tissue slowly to replenish local populations. The replacement is much faster in inflammatory reactions. In addition there is normally in these local populations a certain amount of local replacement. Extirpation of peripheral populations under experimental circumstances may lead to complete replacement from a marrow source. There may be a certain amount of recirculation of peripheral populations; these cells pass mostly to the lungs where they are excreted. The circulating macrophage precursor may be equated in the main with the blood monocyte. It seems likely however that some cells which are usually identified as large lymphocytes may be able to differentiate into macrophages.

The Derivation of Lymph Node Macrophages

The derivation of lymph node macrophages is at present not entirely clear. Undoubtedly within lymph nodes there are some blood derived monocytes and it must be assumed that at least some lymph node macrophages derive therefrom. Also some macrophages may be found in the afferent lymph (Hall et al., 1967; Smith et al., 1970a, b); again it is not known what contribution these make to the static population of macrophages within the lymph node.

It is not so easy to see how sinus macrophages can develop from circulating monocytes; in the rat when a transplantable metastasizing neoplasm is injected into the footpad, there is a proliferation of sinus macrophages within 24 h in the draining lymph node. It is most unlikely that this reaction is tumour specific; it however gives clear evidence of the proliferative potential of sinus macrophages in a model rather similar to human disease (Carr and McGinty, 1973) (Fig. 57).

In this model too, scattered non-lymphoid interstitial cells may be found in mitosis; these often have long processes or may be actually stellate and contain relatively scanty cytoplasmic membranes and a few small lysosomes (Fig. 28). In the same way in animals sensitized to a polysaccharide antigen similar interstitial cells in lymph nodes draining the site of antigen injection show evidence of DNA synthesis (Fig. 29). These cells may be described as reticulum cells; since intermediate forms exist between them and mature macrophages, at least some interstitial macrophages may derive from them.

Chapter Four

MACROPHAGES IN CULTURE

It is not difficult to establish a short-term mixed culture containing a preponderance of macrophages but much harder to obtain macrophages in pure long term culture (Chang, 1964). The culture of macrophages has been reviewed in detail by Jacoby (1965).

In most explants of small pieces of vertebrate tissue cultured in the presence of serum (or "mixed cultures") amoeboid highly motile phagocytic cells are first of all prominent at the edge of the culture, and then outgrow the other cell types in the culture, forming a halo. Whatever the source, once explanted, the cells become structurally and functionally very similar.

Pure cultures of macrophages were first obtained by Carrel and Ebeling (1922) from buffy coats of chicken blood. Here the purity of the culture depends on the alleged "fact" that all the other cells degenerate. Alternatively (Jacoby, 1965) the halo around a piece of chick tissue in culture may be removed and subcultured, though this is technically tricky. This technique is less successful with mammalian tissues than chick but has been used successfully with milk spots (Aronson and Elberg, 1962; Aronson and Shahar, 1965). Perhaps the best way to obtain a pure culture is by washing out a serosal cavity, usually the peritoneal cavity, either in a mammal or chick. Other cells are present but will either degenerate rapidly, as do the polymorphs, or fail to stick to the glass and are washed off with the first change of medium, as are the lymphocytes. Cultures of human peritoneal macrophages have been obtained in this way (Stuart, 1967).

In all of these techniques the macrophages are cultivated on a glass surface; their shape will, of course, be very different from that of the relatively spherical cell obtained by, for example, washing out the peritoneal cavity, but perhaps not very different from the shape of the cell as it lies in the tissue spaces.

The classical description of the macrophage in culture is that of Carrel and Ebeling (1926). The cells studied were cultivated both from blood and from subcutaneous connective tissue. Their most prominent characteristic was the undulating membrane found along the leading edge of the cell as it moved. Unlike fibroblasts they thrived in serum and were relatively resistant to arsenious oxide; these properties are clearly related to those necessary for survival among the hazards of an inflammatory exudate. They enlarged in media rich in serum or when there was much material available from phagocytosis and developed prominent neutral red vacuoles; in starvation, in a poor medium they shrank in size and the neutral red vacuoles decreased in number. Much recent work clearly stems from this paper.

The structure of the macrophages in culture varies with the length of time it has been in culture and, with the source. The phases in its culture have been described (Bennett, 1966) as (1) adherence, (2) spreading and phagocytosis of debris, (3) mitosis and (4) extended culture. With the scanning electron microscope the shape of peritoneal macrophages can be followed during the process of settling on a glass surface; it changes from spherical to a flattened round form and then to a flat stellate form (Carr and Carr, 1970). Very fine protoplasmic processes are extruded during this change (Fig. 35). During prolonged culture the shape may be flattened and approximately circular, elongated or fully extended and may measure 15–80 μm. Stellate forms may sometimes be formed with curious end knobs. When the cell is moving a broad undulating flap-like membrane may act as the leading edge; sometimes two processes may be seen advancing in slightly different directions, each led by a small undulating membrane. Sometimes adjacent cells on a flat surface may apparently adhere to one another so closely as to form a membrane which will strip off the glass as such (Jacoby, 1965). Multinucleate giant cells may form either in these membranes or in their absence (e.g. Goldstein, 1954).

Considerable cytoplasmic detail may often be seen by appropriate staining methods. For instance, vacuoles staining supravitally with neutral red, often lie in a rosette around the cell centre. The distinction made by some early workers between two types of macrophage—the haematogenous monocyte and the tissue clasmatocyte—on the basis of neutral red staining would probably be held now to signify nothing more than a difference between immature and mature versions of the same cell.

Much of the tissue culture work on macrophages has been done on cells derived from serous sacs; there are however differences in behaviour in

inhibited cell on the other hand is smooth without processes. The authors speculate that MIF as well as inhibiting migration is likely to inhibit a wide variety of the cell's metabolic activities. Generally peritoneal macrophages are used; alveolar macrophages however migrate faster (Pollock *et al.*, 1971).

Early workers (see Jacoby, 1965) cast some doubt on the ability of mammalian macrophages to divide in tissue culture but there now seems no doubt that given the right culture conditions they can do so. Macrophages from different sources have different propensities for mitosis *in vitro* (Bennett, 1966). The topic of proliferation of macrophages in general has been discussed in Chapter Three.

It has been thought for many years that macrophages in culture may turn into fibroblasts (Carrel and Ebeling, 1926) under various stimuli. It is indeed true that they can turn into spindle cells similar in appearance to fibroblasts in culture. There is as yet, however, no unequivocal evidence that they can lay down collagen, the only real test of whether a cell is a fibroblast.

Much work on various properties of macrophages has been done in tissue culture, and notably recently on the property of pinocytosis: ingestion of the surrounding fluid medium. This will be discussed under the relevant property rather than under the heading "tissue culture".

The wide variation in shape in macrophages in culture has led several workers to postulate the existence of several types of macrophage and notably to distinguish those which have long spidery processes (e.g. Lewis and Webster, 1921). Stuart (1967) has isolated and cultured human macrophages from a variety of lymphoreticular tissues and has shown (Stuart and Davidson, 1971a, b and c) that after 3–14 days in culture there is a distinct population of cells with long thin processes; these cells contain acid phosphatase and other lysosomal enzymes and also succinate, lactate and malate dehydrogenases. They contain few phagosomes but numerous polyribosomes; while they show close ultrastructural adhesion to one another they do not show contact inhibition of movement. They are less phagocytic for particles than macrophages but more so than fibroblasts. Macrophages tend to cluster round them in culture. Stuart and Davidson (1971c) infer that they may receive antigens from true macrophages *in vitro*, and have christened these cells reticular cells—an unfortunate term in view of the history of confusion in its meaning. There is no absolute evidence of identity between these cells and dendritic macrophages in intact lymphoreticular tissues.

One of the major sources from which these "reticular" cells were cultured was the peritoneal cavity. Fischer *et al.* (1970) have identified a dendritic cell in mouse omentum which is phagocytic for particles and binds antigens. On the other hand numerous workers examining peritoneal cells have failed to identify a separate reticular cell type. There is good evidence (Carr and Carr, 1970) that populations of macrophages which do not contain any elongated cells to start with may rapidly produce them in culture. Stuart and Davidson's interesting work clearly requires further follow up.

Chapter Five

INGESTION BY MACROPHAGES— PHAGOCYTOSIS

The ingestion of foreign material by cells was first clearly described by Metchnikoff though it had been mentioned by several earlier workers. The term phagocytosis initially meant the ingestion of solid foreign material by cells. More recently it has been realized that there are a number of ways in which cells may take in material. As long ago as 1931 Lewis showed that fibroblasts or macrophages in tissue culture would take in microscopically visible droplets of the culture fluid, i.e. pinocytosis. Not long after the introduction of the electron microscope it became apparent that small particles could be ingested in tiny vesicles $0 \cdot 1$ μm or less in diameter; this has been given several names of which perhaps the best was micropinocytosis. The general field of uptake of substances by cells has been reviewed by Jacques (1970). Since the main mechanism used by the macrophage is phagocytosis, this will be discussed first.

The phenomenon of phagocytosis as seen in living cells in tissue culture or in a rabbit's ear chamber is dramatic. The macrophage which has been moving with a flapping ruffle at its leading edge pushes out a process towards the particle and rapidly flows around it. The process of ingestion may take only a few minutes. Once ingested, the material may be totally digested, may persist in the form of an indigestible residue, may actually fill the cell, or if toxic may kill the cell. Another less common form of phagocytosis occurs when the particle is too large for one cell to ingest and several cells flow round it and form a capsule.

The early literature on phagocytosis was reviewed by Mudd *et al.* (1934), Berry and Spies (1949) and Hirsch (1965). Phagocytosis may be initiated by interfacial surface tension forces (Fenn, 1921) but is energy dependent (Baldridge and Gerard, 1934) and dependent on an environment suitable for living processes in terms of ionic concentration and temperature. While in some systems phagocytosis can proceed in the absence of protein in the medium, in general it is stimulated by the presence of protein and in the case of bacteria by specific opsonic antibodies. Much of the early work was done with polymorphs but the basic process is similar in the macrophage.

Mudd *et al.* (1934) pointed out the similarity between the way in which a phagocyte spreads on a surface and the way in which it spreads on a particle (phagocytosis). Macrophages being more viscous and less deformable spread on surfaces less readily and spread more slowly than polymorphs.

It was early recognized that macrophages perform an important function in the phagocytosis of dead tissue. For instance Deno (1936) described the removal of debris from the placental site; the placental site becomes transformed into a mass of macrophages which persist for a considerable time.

Phagocytosis in the Amoeba

Phagocytosis has been studied in great detail in the amoeba, mainly because amoebae are large and fairly easy to experiment with. Some account will therefore be given of phagocytosis in the amoeba largely as a pointer to how little is known about the way in which macrophages phagocytose.

The ultrastructure of the process has been well illustrated by Christensen and Marshall (1965). Contact between the amoeba and its prey induces an outsurge of cytoplasm which lifts the plasmalemma, probably the point of initial contact between prey and amoeba. The cytoplasm deep to the membrane here is probably in the gel state, and motionless. Next the lips of the food cup move together and the approximated membranes overlap and fuse. Deep to the food cup is a specialized region of channels and small vesicles which may be related to digestion, though the precise nature of this relation is at present not clear.

A detailed and co-ordinated study of phagocytosis by the amoeba has been published by Korn and Weisman (1967). These workers studied in a precise way the uptake of polystyrene beads of various sizes. Provided that osmotic conditions were correct there was no need for the presence of any specific organic molecule. Uptake of particles was highly selective in that up to 30% of the polystyrene beads could be abstracted from the fluid environment without ingestion of any significant quantity of radioactive glucose from the environment. Beads more than $1 \cdot 3$ μm in diameter were ingested singly whereas beads less than $0 \cdot 6$ μm in diameter lingered on the cell membrane till a little packet of beads accumulated. This was then ingested. Obviously during this process there is a large scale utilization of cell membrane substance. Little change occurs however in the total volume of the amoeba. There must be therefore either rapid synthesis or rapid translocation of membrane substance. Phagocytic vesicles have been isolated by ultracentrifugation both as vesicles and as open sheets. The whole process of ingestion is inhibited by substances which inhibit glycolysis.

There is a need for similarly exact and extensive studies of phagocytosis as it occurs in mammalian cells.

Quantitation

Numerous attempts have been made to quantitate the phenomenon of phagocytosis mainly on the basis of counting either the percentage of cells in a population which can phagocytose, or the number of particles ingested by individual cells. These subjective assessments are subject to numerous pitfalls notably the difficulty in assessing microscopically whether a given particle is or is not within a cell. One of the best of the many counting techniques is that of Vaughan (1965) in which known numbers of phagocytes and particles are deposited on a test membrane and allowed to interact for a known period.

More recent techniques have involved the use of radioactive labelled bacteria (Downey and Diedrich, 1968) and quantitative counting of the radioactivity, or the use of medium containing radioactive albumin (Chang, 1969). The fluid medium enters the phagocytes with the particles during phagocytosis; if ^{131}I labelled serum albumin is added to the medium the amount of this taken up by the cells will be a measure of phagocytosis. One of the commonest test objects used in studies of phagocytosis has been the red blood cell; phagocytosis of red blood cells can be measured fairly readily by measuring the amount of intracellular haemoglobin spectrophotometrically. A difficulty lies in getting rid of the extracellular red blood cells. A particularly useful technique of this type is that of Morita and Perkins (1965), who found that once red blood cells had been ingested they were protected against mild osmotic shock. The number of red blood cells ingested in a test system of macrophages could therefore be assessed by subjecting the cells to mild osmotic shock and then estimating their haemoglobin content, which would now give an accurate representation of the number of red blood cells phagocytosed.

The Stages of Phagocytosis

Phagocytosis can be divided into attachment, ingestion and digestion. The result of interaction between macrophage and particle (whether inorganic or bacterial) may vary widely. Thus the macrophage may kill the bacterium and only degenerate fragments of the latter persist within the cytoplasm; the converse may happen, or the two may live in symbiosis. The precursor of phagocytosis may be chemotaxis—the reaction whereby the direction of locomotion of cells is determined by chemical substances in the environment (McCutcheon, 1946). Since this is, strictly speaking, an *in vitro* phenomenon, it has been described in Chapter Four.

Attachment

With the phase contrast or scanning electron microscopes, the surface of the macrophage can be seen to be formed into irregular flaps and ruffles; at high resolution with the transmission electron microscope the surface zone can be seen to be composed of a superficial cell coat 8–16 nm thick of acidic mucosubstance, the cell coat, lying on the outer surface of the bilamellar unit membrane and lightly adherent to it. Deep to this lies a cytoplasmic zone notably free of organelles; in this zone a few small fibrils can occasionally be made out in favourable sections. With the ruthenium red staining technique a rather ill-defined pattern of densities is visible on the cell surface. It seems possible that this may be related in some way to a discontinuous arrangement of antigenic determinants on cell surfaces. Aoki *et al.* (1969) have studied the distribution of various antigens on cell surfaces by staining them with the appropriate antibody labelled with ferritin. In the mouse cells studied by these workers the antigens studied occurred discontinuously on the cell surface; the distribution of antigen-containing areas was characteristic for each cell. Of the antigens studied the only one present on macrophages was the H2 antigen—the main blood group compatibility antigen of the species. There was quite a striking difference between peritoneal macrophages and "reticular cells" from spleen, lymph nodes or thymus. The latter cells had H2 antigen over all of their surfaces except the tips of processes while peritoneal macrophages had the antigen only over scattered patches on the surface. This means firstly that the surface of a macrophage is heterogeneous despite the relatively homogeneous appearance seen in conventional electron micrographs. Secondly it implies that considerable differences may exist between macrophage surfaces from one site to another. Closely related to these heterogeneities is the problem of the existence of cytophilic antibody and of globulin receptors on macrophage surfaces.

Cytophilic antibodies are immunoglobulins, usually but not always IgG, attached to cell surfaces and probably in equilibrium with globulins in the surrounding fluid (Boyden and Sorkin, 1961; Boyden, 1961, 1962, 1964; Berken and Benacerraf, 1966). Cytophilic antibody may be attached to the macrophage surface by a receptor which can sometimes but not always be detached by digestion with trypsin and which may contain SH groups and a phospholipid.

It seems likely that specific receptors on macrophage membranes may initiate phagocytosis. If loosely bound these might be regarded as cytophilic antibody, while if tightly bound they might be part of the surface muco-protein complex.

Various views have been put forward on the nature of these receptors. Lay and Nussenzweig (1968, 1969) have demonstrated three separate receptors, for complement, IgM and IgG, varying in sensitivity to trypsinization and dependence on local ionic concentration. Receptors for cytophilic antibody are phospholipoprotein (Davey and Asherson, 1966) and contain SH groups (Howard and Benacerraf, 1966). Those for IgG may actually resemble complement in structure (Hess and Luscher, 1970). The receptors for opsonized bacteria are protein in structure (Allen and Cook, 1970).

Some topographical localization for receptors comes from the work of Lo Buglio *et al.* (1967) who showed receptors for IgG on the surface of human monocytes and macrophages and pointed out that phagocytosis was initiated at multiple regularly spaced points of adhesion where (presumably) receptors are localized. Rabinowitch (1968, 1970) suggested that there might be at least two kinds of receptors, one for denatured particles and one for antibodies and perhaps a third for reactions in which complement was involved. There is need for further work on the topographical localization of all these receptors.

The requirements for attachment vary from system to system; for instance attachment of effete red blood cells is dependent on a cytophilic antibody on the macrophage surface (Vaughan and Boyden, 1964; Boyden, 1964). Attachment of glutaraldehyde-fixed red blood cells to macrophages is temperature dependent but proceeds independently of serum or divalent cations; attachment is abolished by trypsinization. The presence of serum and divalent cations in the medium is, however, necessary for ingestion of the red blood cells; attachment is promoted by specific antisera (Rabinowitch *et al.*, 1967a, b, c). The initial step in particle-cell contact may be formation of calcium bridges between particle and cell (Metzger and Casarett, 1969).

The attachment phase of the ingestion of bacteria has been studied by Allen and Cook (1970) and the pattern shown to be similar to that of red cells. A macroglobulin from calf serum acted as opsonin. The surface receptor for the opsonized bacteria was found to be sensitive to proteolytic enzymes, and is therefore probably protein in nature.

The phenomenon of recognition of material as foreign must be regarded as occurring when the particle first adheres to the cell surface. If it sticks an irreversible series of events resulting in ingestion occurs. Therefore discrimination between foreign and autochthonous material may be said to occur according to whether material does or does not stick.

This may depend however on the presence of a suitable layer of opsonizing protein. Pisano *et al.* (1970) have shown that whereas the plasma of normal human subjects contains opsonin for the ingestion of a gelatinized lipid emulsion, that of cancer patients does not. They infer from this a failure of "recognition" in cancer patients and postulate that this may be related to their disease.

A good example of the discriminatory power of macrophages was given by Stuart *et al.* (1967). When mouse macrophages were grown *in vitro* in human AB serum they readily ingested human RBC sensitized with for instance Anti A serum. In this system they would recognize and phagocytose old but not fresh RBC, showing fairly sensitive discrimination.

There have been few studies of the recognition and phagocytosis of degenerate autologous elements; Stuart *et al.* (1969) showed that in mouse typhoid where hepatic epithelial cells are damaged, macrophages may protrude processes into them and segregate and phagocytose mitochondria.

Ingestion

The actual mechanism of the cytoplasmic movements involved in the ingestion phase of phagocytosis is obscure but on a superficial level the ultrastructural features have been examined in some detail; they vary with the relative size of particle and phagocyte and with the mobility of the phagocyte. Where small particles such as carbon, impinge on the wall of relatively immobile cells like pulmonary alveolar macrophages they are swept by active ruffling movements of cell membrane into vacuoles which then pass deep into the cell (Karrer, 1960).

When a macrophage in tissue culture ingests a red blood cell, a flap of macrophage cytoplasm protrudes round and finally covers the red blood cell, meeting another similar process on the other side (Fig. 39). The process of phagocytosis of red blood cells is discussed in Chapter Nine. When macrophages in suspension are phagocytosing lipid globules, cytoplasmic processes are protruded and at the same time a deep indentation of cytoplasm forms, enclosing several globules (Fig. 40).

Where the phagocyte is firmly fixed, for instance the Kupffer cell, and is phagocytosing bacteria passing by in the blood stream, finger-like or flap-like processes of cytoplasm are extended into the blood stream to trap the bacteria (Horn et al., 1969). These processes are composed almost entirely of ectoplasm and do not contain lysosomes or other organelles.

A curious feature of the contact zone between phagocyte and bacterium or other particles is the presence of an area of increased cytoplasmic density just below the cell membrane (North and Mackaness, 1963b; Horn et al., 1969; Lo Buglio et al., 1967). The dense area contains small granules and sometimes small filaments similar to those seen in the cytoplasmic flaps of macrophages which are not obviously engaged in phagocytosis.

Where the mass of material to be phagocytosed is larger than the phagocyte the process of ingestion is somewhat different. This situation arises in the case of the osteoclast (see Chapter Ten) or where macrophages have to deal with such objects as masses of lipid or artificially introduced foreign material (Gusek, 1959, 1964; Carr, 1962; Curran and Clark, 1964). Macrophages become very closely apposed to the foreign substance and adherent to one another by tightly interlocking cell processes; the cytoplasm next to the foreign material is entirely ectoplasmic and free of organelles. Often no space can be resolved between the macrophage membrane and the foreign body. Particles of the foreign substance (Figs 37 and 38) appear within the phagocyte; the mechanism of this is not entirely clear. Sometimes as in the case of the osteoclast many fine cytoplasmic processes are protruded into the foreign substance, presumably breaking it up. There is a possibility that lysosomal enzymes may be secreted outside the macrophage, though this is by no means certain (Curran and Clark, 1964).

Shirahama et al. (1971) have analysed in an interesting way the interaction between peritoneal macrophages and aggregates of material of various sizes. Where the aggregate is less than 2 μm in size the macrophage treats it as a small particle and wraps processes round it. Where the mass measures more than 10 μm several macrophages appose to it and intrude small cytoplasmic projections. With masses in between 2 and 10 μm in size, single macrophages attempt to ingest it but also attempt to intrude processes, that is the process of ingestion is intermediate.

The crux of the process of ingestion is cytoplasmic movement. Clearly several forms of movement can be involved. Firstly there may be movement of a cytoplasmic flap or ruffle; this can be observed by phase contrast microscopy of living cells. With the electron microscope fine fibrils can be seen in the centre of some such processes. Secondly there may be a shearing movement of a surface layer of cytoplasm over the rest of the cell; the surface layer of ectoplasm certainly contains fine filaments. Thirdly there is undoubted movement of phagocytic vacuoles; no credible ultrastructural basis for this has been observed. In none of these instances can the metabolic changes which have been shown to occur be satisfactorily related to the morphological findings.

In a system where attachment and ingestion of glutaraldehyde fixed RBC are dissociated, ingestion is stimulated by the presence of divalent cations, serum and in particular by specific antisera, notably IgG (Rabinowitch, 1967a, b, c). Macrophages previously treated with staphylococci will ingest more RBC (Rabinowitch and Gary, 1968) due both to an increase in the proportion of cells which are phagocytically active and to an increase in the phagocytic ability of individual macrophages.

Digestion

After the initial ingestion in a membranous vesicle, the phagosome fuses with one or several lysosomes containing acid phosphatase and other lysosomal enzymes. Views vary on the actual morphology of the primary lysosomes. North and Mackaness (1963a) illustrated them as small electron lucent vesicles; other workers (Carr, 1968b; Horn et al., 1969; Leake and Myrvik, 1968, 1970) have depicted small membrane bound bodies with electron dense cores as fusing with phagosomes and regarded these as primary lysosomes. It is likely that the structures depicted are the same; the latter workers have in the main used uranium staining, which renders the protein core of lysosomes electron dense. It seems likely that as well as primary lysosomes fusing with phagosomes, secondary lysosomes containing some previously ingested material may do so (Fig. 41). The largest secondary lysosomes, however, are inert and do not incorporate significant amounts of foreign material.

The end product of digestion, the residual body, is a large irregular electron dense mass often containing laminated myelin whorls presumably phospholipid, and sometimes ferritin from breakdown of red blood cells. Completely indigestible material such as carbon may persist unaltered, while bacteria may survive and either kill the macrophage or live in symbiosis with it. For instance in experimental leprosy apparently intact bacilli may be found lying in vacuoles surrounded by lysosomal material, in an apparently intact cell many months after infection (Allen *et al.*, 1965). Similarly in infection with *Brucella*, bacteria may persist within the cell for a long time (Karlsbad *et al.*, 1964).

The lysosomal enzymes of macrophages have been studied by Cohn and Wiener (1963a, b) in cell fractions obtained by ultracentrifugation. A fraction composed largely of macrophage cytoplasmic granules contained acid phosphatase, lysozyme, acid ribonuclease, β-glucuronidase, cathepsin and lipase; after phagocytosis these enzymes were demonstrable in the soluble cytoplasmic fraction—that is they had passed from one cytoplasmic compartment to another. While a complete co-ordinated morphological and chemical study has yet to be done, this almost certainly represents passage from lysosome to phagosome.

Cohn (1963a, b) studied the fate of bacteria in phagocytic cells. The bacteria studied (*B. subtilis* and *E. coli*) were killed rapidly: 95% in 1 h and degraded extensively within 2 h. There was no significant incorporation of low molecular weight products from the bacterium into the structure of the phagocyte. While the presence of inhibitors of glycolysis (iodoacetate or arsenite) blocked the ingestion stage of phagocytosis, it did not affect subsequent digestion. It seems that while ingestion is energy dependent, subsequent digestion is not. It is interesting however that Hor *et al.* (1969) found that fusion of phagosome and lysosome occurred readily *in vivo*, but not in the presumably inferior environment of an *in vitro* experiment. Both ingestion and digestion are relatively radio-resistant (Perkins *et al.*, 1966).

Axline and Cohn (1970) showed that *in vitro* phagocytosis of red blood cells induced formation of lysosomal enzymes. The critical step in phagocytosis which is responsible for triggering synthesis of lysosomal enzymes is probably not ingestion or fusion of phagosome and lysosome, since there is no formation of lysosomal enzymes in response to ingestion of

indigestible materials like starch or polystyrene particles. It seems likely
therefore that it is the actual process of digestion. Digestion is inhibited
by colchicine treatment (Lockard *et al.*, 1971).

The earliest report on the metabolic changes occurring during phagocytosis was that of Baldridge and Gerard (1933). They incubated dog
leucocytes in Ringer's solution with added serum and found a burst of
"extra respiration" after addition of bacteria to the suspension. It took
many years however before the view that phagocytosis required energy
gained general acceptance. Because polymorphs are more readily obtained,
most of the studies which led to the acceptance of this view were done
with polymorphonuclear leucocytes (see review by Karnovsky, 1962).
The metabolism of polymorphs, peritoneal macrophages and alveolar
macrophages was studied in some detail by Oren *et al.* (1963). Alveolar
macrophages have a much higher respiratory activity than the other two
types of cells. Polymorphs and peritoneal macrophages convert most of
their glucose to lactate by anaerobic pathways. Uptake of oxygen was
increased when the cells were incubated with particles; this increase was
well marked in the case of alveolar macrophages. On addition of metabolic
inhibitors polymorphs and mononuclears were found to phagocytose
adequately when aerobic respiration was stopped. Inhibition of glycolysis
however stopped phagocytosis.

The stage of phagocytosis at which energy is consumed is probably
actual ingestion. Rabinowitch (1967a) showed that initial adhesion was
not energy dependent. Cohn (1963a, b) examined the uptake of isotopically
labelled bacteria by macrophages and showed that inhibitors of glycolysis
blocked actual uptake of the bacteria but did not inhibit degradation of
the bacteria once ingested. The initial step of degradation of the bacteria
was liberation of the pool of small molecular weight components in the
bacterium followed by degradation of the high molecular weight components.

Reticuloendothelial Clearance

The reticuloendothelial system is able to clear both inert particles and
bacteria by phagocytosis from the bloodstream (see Cappell, 1929). The
clearance of relatively coarse colloidal suspensions such as carbon has been
studied in great detail (see Stuart, 1970; Stiffel *et al.*, 1970 for review).
Under standard experimental conditions carbon suspensions are cleared

in a very regular way and have been held to give some measure of the overall activity of the reticuloendothelial system. The prior administration of various substances has been shown to stimulate or depress clearance of carbon. For instance, yeast extracts, zymosan and glucan stimulate clearance (Riggi and Diluzio, 1961) as do oestrogens (see Vernon Roberts, 1970) and the glycerol esters of fatty acids (Stuart *et al.*, 1960) while the alkyl esters of fatty acids depress clearance (Stuart *et al.*, 1960).

It was supposed initially that the results of carbon clearance tests reflected a fairly simple clearance of particles from the circulation by a fairly homogeneous population of macrophages; it has become clear more recently that matters are not so simple and that clearance tests do not simply represent macrophage function. For instance Gabrieli *et al.* (1967) showed that variations in binding of carbon on to a plasma component affect clearance and Jeunet *et al.* (1967, 1969) related failure of clearance in part to exhaustion of plasma opsonin. When the clearance of a colloid is examined ultrastructurally it is evident that it is dependent not only on uptake by macrophages but on the rate of leakage between endothelial cells and out of the circulation (Carr, 1968b). Singer *et al.* (1969) have shown that carbon particles may be trapped by platelet aggregates. Nevertheless there is evidence that alteration in macrophage function may be involved in variations in clearance rate. For instance glucan and zymosan produce cellular proliferation and also make the Kupffer cells swell into the lumen of the hepatic sinusoid (Ashworth *et al.*, 1963; Nicolescu and Rouiller, 1967). Emulsions of glyceryl trioleate produce a surface stimulation of peritoneal cells and may have a similar effect on Kupffer cells (Carr, 1967b). Conversely thorotrast and cortisone block the surface attachment phase of phagocytosis (Wiener *et al.*, 1967) and ethyl palmitate actually destroys macrophages (Stuart, 1960).

Few studies of reticuloendothelial clearance have involved adequate ultrastructural and quantitative investigation. A recent thorough investigation has been carried out on the clearance of carbon and latex particles by Singer *et al.* (1969); and Adlersberg *et al.* (1969). There were significant differences in clearance of these two substances, for instance latex clearance was independent of dose while carbon clearance was inversely proportionate to dose. More that 90% of both colloids was removed from the circulation within 5 min. Phagocytosis of latex involved coating of the particles and indentation of the cell surface, while phagocytosis of carbon involved formation of channels on the cell surface. There was clear evidence of extraphagocytic distribution of considerable quantities of colloid and of trapping of aggregates of particles by platelets in the spleen. These findings clearly indicate that colloid clearance tests are affected by a complex set of variables and that any systematic variation in colloid clearance cannot be reasonably represented as a single entity such as reticuloendothelial function. Moreover such colloid clearance is not necessarily related to successful phagocytosis and destruction of bacteria, the basis of resistance to disease.

Chapter Six

INGESTION BY MACROPHAGES— PINOCYTOSIS AND MICROPINOCYTOSIS

While phagocytosis is the most characteristic way in which macrophages ingest material, they may like other cells ingest material in other ways. An important demonstration of two patterns of ingestion was given by Gordon and King (1960), who showed that fibroblasts in tissue culture took up carmine particles by an energy dependent process but thorotrast by a non-energy dependent process, probably merely physical adsorption. The uptake of lipid and lipoprotein aggregates of various sizes by macrophages *in vitro* was studied by Casley-Smith and Day (1966). They showed that cholesterol and corn oil particles 50 nm to 5 nm in diameter passed into cells by way of large vesicles 1 μm or larger in size, which formed either by indentation of the surface of the macrophage or by the protrusion and fusion of pseudopodia. These large particles were taken up much more rapidly at 37°C than at 4°C. Lipoprotein particles on the other hand entered the cells almost as rapidly at 0°C as at 37°C, in small (approximately 50 nm) vesicles. A further study by Casley-Smith (1969) investigated the energy requirements for the uptake of various particles ranging in size from bacteria to ferritin. Large particles (larger than 0·1 μm) entered the cell in large vesicles (0·1–5 μm in diameter). Small particles (less than 50 nm) in diameter enter the cell usually in small vesicles (approximately 70 nm diameter). These may later coalesce to form large vesicles. Entry in large vesicles whether of large particles or of groups of small ones was inhibited by the metabolic inhibitors used. Since the inhibitors used (dinitrophenol, sodium cyanide, sodium fluoride, colchicine and iodoacetic acid) were used in rather high doses, precise inferences could not be made about the metabolic pathways on which uptake was dependent. But the conclusion seems firm: uptake in large vesicles is dependent on cellular metabolism. The initial adsorption on the other hand is not similarly dependent; likewise uptake in small vesicles and the subsequent fusion of these into large vesicles is not energy dependent.

Uptake within small vesicles is best described as micropinocytosis. There was until recently little evidence that this happened in macrophages to any significant extent *in vivo*. Han *et al.* (1970) have shown that lymph node macrophages take up ferritin *in vitro* in small vesicles. These later coalesce to form large vacuoles (Fig. 43). It appears from the micrographs of these authors that small vesicles may form either by invagination of surface membrane or by protrusion of tiny pseudopodia (though they do not comment on these possible variations in mechanism).

It is not certain to what extent the chemical composition of a substance, as opposed to the physical size of the particles into which it is dispersed, affects the mode of its uptake. In particular there is some evidence that in at least some instances proteins may be taken up by ultrastructurally distinct mechanisms.

The general field of protein uptake by cells was surveyed by Ryser (1968). It is now accepted that many cells can take up intact proteins at relatively low rates and without much energy consumption; absorption is enhanced by polybasic compounds. Some proteins are taken up much more readily than others, cationic macromolecules of large molecular weights most readily of all. Once they have been ingested proteins are often rapidly broken down.

It was suggested by Roth and Porter (1964) on the basis of their findings on the uptake of yolk protein by insect oocytes that certain vesicles covered with a layer of fine bristles or spikes, so-called "coated vesicles", were responsible for the uptake of protein. Friend and Farquar (1967) showed that two distinct populations of coated vesicles existed in the cells of the rat vas deferens. Both types of vesicle had a coat of radially arranged bristles extending from the outer leaflet of the limiting membrane; each bristle was 15–20 nm long. The small vesicles some 75 nm in diameter served as primary lysosomes to carry hydrolytic enzymes from the Golgi region, while the larger vesicles, some 100 nm in diameter served for the absorption of artificially administered peroxidase; coated vesicles exist in macrophages (Carr, 1968a). Their formation has been studied by Shira-hama and Cohen (1970) who examined the uptake of human amyloid by mouse peritoneal macrophages *in vitro*. Dense areas were found just below the cell membrane in relation to aggregates of amyloid in contact with the cell membrane. These dense areas are 30–50 nm thick and extend over

200–800 nm of the cell membrane. A credible set of images was presented which suggested that these structures developed into invaginations which in their turn became typical coated vesicles.

A variant of micropinocytosis has been described in Kupffer cells (Toro *et al.*, 1962; Orci *et al.*, 1967; Matter *et al.*, 1968). After stimulation with such widely different stimuli as indian ink, tetracycline, streptozotocine and partial hepatectomy, tubular invaginations 0·1 μm wide appear on the vascular pole of the cells. Three dimensional reconstruction shows that these in fact form an intricate labyrinth of tubes and clefts with multiple openings to the extracellular space. Many coated vesicles were found in the cytoplasm adjacent to these clefts; about one in ten of these coated vesicles actually communicated with the clefts. It has been suggested that this type of complex micropinocytotic system may be associated with protein absorption but there is no very good evidence for this.

The above discussion refers to uptake of large or small aggregates of solid material in either large or very small vesicles. In addition (at least *in vitro*) macrophages can take up considerable amounts of fluid by pinocytosis (Fig. 42). This should be regarded as a phenomenon distinct from phagocytosis (Rabinovitch, 1970). It has not been shown clearly to occur in the living animal and its significance is therefore uncertain.

Pinocytosis as it occurs in mouse peritoneal macrophages has been extensively studied by Cohn and his colleagues (1965, 1966, 1967, reviewed 1968, 1970). When mouse macrophages are cultured in the presence of serum, notably new born calf serum, numerous phase lucent pinocytic vesicles appear. These have a half life of 19–29 min; at the same time there is an accumulation of dense granules and the cells can be shown biochemically to produce cathepsin, β-glucuronidase and acid phosphatase. Pinocytosis is blocked by a wide variety of metabolic inhibitors—e.g. sodium fluoride, cyanide, dinitrophenol and puromycin, probably in a rather non-specific way. The whole process of pinocytosis and accumulation of hydrolytic enzymes can be reversed by putting the cells into a medium of low serum content. Numerous factors induce pinocytosis (Cohn and Parks, 1967a, b, c). Among them are proteins with isoelectric points of pH 5 or less, fatty acids, acidic mucosubstances, DNA and RNA. Anionic substances stimulate pinocytosis better than cationic substances and the stimulant effect increases with molecular weight. Spectacular stimulation of pinocytosis is produced by adenosine triphosphate, which also stimulates spreading on glass. Potent stimulation may be produced immunologically; a macroglobulin in bovine serum is potent in stimulating pinocytosis by mouse macrophages. It is probably an antibody against macrophage cell membrane. There seems little doubt that *in vitro*, pinocytosis increases formation of hydrolytic enzymes within the cell; the mechanism of this is obscure.

The fate of labelled protein pinocytosed by macrophages *in vitro* has been studied in some detail (Ehrenreich and Cohn, 1968, 1969; Cohn and Ehrenreich, 1969). The major labelled degradation product of digestion of serum albumin was monoiodotyrosine. Similar results were obtained in the case of digestion of haemoglobin. It therefore seems very likely that *in vitro* macrophages can degrade proteins to the level of amino-acids, probably within the lysosomes; it is not certain whether similar degradations can occur *in vivo*.

The uptake and metabolism of carbohydrates by macrophages *in vitro* has been studied by Cohn and Ehrenreich (1969) and Ehrenreich and Cohn (1969). The ingestion of sucrose leads to the development of large phase-lucent vacuoles. The molecule apparently cannot escape from the vacuole since it is of too high a molecular weight, while the macrophages do not possess the appropriate enzymes to break it down. When invertase, the enzyme which breaks down sucrose, is added to the culture, the large vacuoles disappear. Monosaccharides having a molecular weight below 220 do not generally induce vacuolation, while disaccharides, with a molecular weight of 300 or more do induce vacuolation. Most peptides do not induce vacuolation. Synthetic dextro-compounds with a molecular radius above 0·4 nm (that is too high to pass through the vacuole membrane) do however induce vacuolation.

Chapter Seven

THE MACROPHAGE IN REPAIR, INFLAMMATION AND THE IMMUNE RESPONSE

Macrophages participate in the defence of the mammalian organism in a number of ways. They remove debris during tissue involution and repair; they destroy micro-organisms by phagocytosis, often as part of an organized extravascular aggregate of inflammatory cells or granuloma. They may take up and process antigens. They may kill antigenically deviant cells, notably neoplastic cells and they may actively secrete various substances: lysozyme, interferon and pyrogen. Phagocytosis has already been considered and secretion by macrophages will be described in Chapter Eight. The defensive functions of the macrophage have been reviewed by Shands (1967), Mackaness and Blanden (1967), Dannenberg (1968) and Nelson (1969).

Involution and Repair

During repair and reorganization of tissues, macrophages ingest and digest fragments of dead cells and altered collagen. The need for this may occur during resorption of an organ which is involuting for physiological reasons—for example the placental site at the end of pregnancy or the mammary gland at the end of lactation. Or it may occur during resorption of damaged tissue in a wound or an area of ischaemic necrosis.

Situations where involution has been studied cytochemically or with the electron microscope include the involution of the uterus post partum (Lobel and Deane, 1962), the resorption of hair follicles (Parakkal, 1969a, b), the involution of lymphoid tissue (Anton and Brandes, 1969), the involution of the mammary gland at the end of lactation (Helminen and Ericsson, 1968a, b; Helminen *et al.*, 1968) and the resorption of the tadpole

77

tail (Weber, 1963). In these situations numerous large macrophages rich in acid phosphatase and other lysosomal enzymes are present; fragments of cell debris are found in secondary lysosomes within these cells. There is some dispute about the mechanism of breakdown of collagen. Parakkal (1969a, b) demonstrated numerous collagen fibres within phagocytic vacuoles inside macrophages. Some of these vesicles also contained acid phosphatase. It appeared therefore that the collagen was being broken down within cells. Kajikawa *et al.* (1970) on the other hand have studied the resorption of collagen in a granuloma produced by subcutaneous injection of carrageenin. Studies with the ultracentrifuge showed that collagenase was present in the same fraction as acid phosphatase. Electron microscopy showed small vesicles containing acid phosphatase near the surface of macrophages; fragmented collagen was seen outside macrophages, but little recognizable collagen within them. The inference from these studies was that the macrophages secreted an enzyme which broke down collagen extracellularly.

The presence of macrophages in healing wounds has been recognized for a long time; their function is the phagocytosis of tissue "debris". Ross and Benditt (1962) and Ross and Odland (1968) illustrated their ultra-structure in studies of wound repair in the guinea-pig and in man. Mono-cytes with poorly developed endoplasmic reticulum enter the wound from the blood stream. As the lesion develops they ingest fibrin, serum protein and other debris and eventually contain numerous large membrane-bounded electron dense bodies. During their development into active macrophages there is an increase in endoplasmic reticulum, probably related to the formation of hydrolytic enzymes.

Ghani (1969) has studied at the light microscope level the organization of experimentally induced mural thrombi; in this situation too, circulating mononuclear cells develop into macrophages and ingest and remove thrombus. From this survey of the role of the macrophage in the resorption of debris it is clear that macrophages can ingest and digest dead cells and altered collagen. It is not clear what are the alterations in an inert substance, collagen, which trigger phagocytosis by macrophages. It seems possible that macrophages can secrete enzymes which cause collagen breakdown.

The important function of the macrophage in infections with bacteria, fungi and viruses is of course phagocytosis. (See Chapter Five). This occurs either as clearance of blood or lymph by fixed macrophages, or in the interstitial tissues. The clearance of bacteria by fixed macrophages has been extensively reviewed by Howard (1961); it is on the whole less efficient than the clearance of circulating inert particles, probably because in a population of bacteria a few are resistant to phagocytosis, possibly due to surface charge. Clearance of bacteria may be expedited by the presence of circulating antibodies which coat the bacteria, or by prior stimulation of the reticuloendothelial system with any of a large number of materials which induce non-specific maturation of macrophages. There is not always a relationship between increased clearance of bacteria and increased cellular function of macrophages, nor between either and clinical resistance to disease.

When bacteria gain access to interstitial tissue only a few local tissue histiocytes are available. It is therefore necessary that there be large scale migration of monocytes from the blood stream, maturation of monocytes into macrophages in the tissues, immobilization of these macrophages within the tissues and probably increased production of monocytes at source.

The migration of monocytes occurs contemporaneously with that of polymorphs; unlike the polymorphs the monocytes survive and mature. Often if an inflammatory lesion becomes chronic large numbers of lymphocytes, macrophages and other inflammatory cells cluster together in focal aggregates known as granulomata. It seems likely that the immobilization of macrophages in a granuloma is due to protein factors or lymphokines, generated on contact between antigen and sensitized lymphocytes (Dumonde et al., 1969. See reviews by Mackaness and Blanden, 1967; Dannenberg, 1968; Stuart, 1970).

The provision of sufficient monocytes to mount an inflammatory response probably requires an increase in output. Willoughby et al. (1967) have shown that when dead tubercle bacilli emulsified in oil (Freund's adjuvant) are injected into lymph nodes there is an increase in the number of circulating monocytes. A similar increase can be induced by injections of serum from animals whose lymph nodes have been injected in this way. These observations suggest that there may be a monocytogenic hormone produced in lymphoid tissue which stimulates monocyte production.

The role of macrophages in virus diseases has been reviewed by Mims (1964b). It seems that viruses are taken up by macrophages in various parts of the body. They may be destroyed intracellularly, may persist, or may kill the cell. The actual uptake of the virus may occur by micropinocytosis or by phagocytosis of groups of virus particles often along with cellular debris (Aronow et al., 1964; Friend et al., 1969).

The fate of bacteria once they are ingested by phagocytes has an important effect on the outcome of the disease. Thus the common pathogenic cocci do not survive within macrophages. Such organisms as *Myco-bacterium tuberculosis*, *Brucella abortus* and *Salmonella typhi* may survive within macrophages. A few bacteria like *Mycobacterium leprae* are obligatory intracellular parasites and can proliferate only within cell cytoplasm. Protozoa, e.g. the various plasmodia of malaria, and leishmania of kala-azar, and some fungi can also survive and multiply within macrophages. In Whipple's disease, macrophages laden with unidentified bacteria infiltrate the small intestinal mucosa (Cohen, 1964; Roberts *et al.*, 1970).

Macrophages in Granulomata

A common pattern in chronic inflammation is for large numbers of cells to aggregate in groups or clusters. This is known as a granuloma. In a typical granuloma there are numerous lymphocytes, plasma cells and monocytes; the macrophages are larger with indented nuclei and frilly margins, or actual, visible, individual processes. They may contain basophilic granules. Some are even larger with poorly staining cytoplasm; these may resemble the cells of surface epithelia and are often described as epithelioid cells. In addition there are some very large cells with numerous nuclei, giant cells. Granulomatous lesions commonly show areas of necrosis and fibrous tissue is often laid down at the periphery.

The macrophages within a granuloma have a similar cytochemical pattern to those elsewhere; they tend to be mature cells rich in hydrolytic enzymes—including acid phosphatase, β-glucuronidase, aminopeptidase and non-specific esterase (Gedigk and Bontke, 1957). In the granuloma induced by the seaweed extract carrageenin (Monis *et al.*, 1968), as to be expected, considerable levels of acid phosphatase, aminopeptidase and several oxidative enzymes were present; the interesting point however was that the macrophages contained high levels of galactosidase, but little glucosidase or glucurunidase. It seems likely that this represents specifically induced enzyme synthesis.

The ultrastructure of macrophages in granulomata has been studied by various groups (Gusek, 1959, 1964; Gusek and Naumann, 1959; Pernis *et al.*, 1966; Carr, 1962; Bonicke *et al.*, 1963; Davis, 1963a, b, 1964; Policard *et al.*, 1965; Dumont and Sheldon, 1965; Galindo and Imaeda, 1966; Adam 1966; see also review by Epstein, 1967). The component macrophages vary widely in size and are often very large; adjacent macrophages are held together by interdigitating membranes (Gusek, 1964; Adam, 1966) and sometimes by desmosomes. Most of these cells are mature and contain numerous lysosomes, usually with a core which is highly electron dense and sometimes paracrystalline; this presumably represents close packed lysosomal enzyme protein. Some of these bodies have tubular or hourglass shaped profiles. Other less electron dense inclusions are visible in the cells of many granulomata, e.g. those of tuberculosis and sarcoidosis (Dumont and Sheldon, 1965; Wanstrup and Christensen, 1966; Williams *et al.*, 1970). The significance of these is not certain (Figs 44 and 45).

The term "epithelioid" cell is sometimes used to describe a large mature macrophage. Elias and Epstein (1968) in a study of the granuloma induced by the injection of beryllium have put forward the view that "epithelioid" cells are a type of cell, peculiar to sensitized subjects and derived directly from monocytes and not from beryllium laden macrophages. Such cells retain a prominent nucleolus even when very large and have only a moderate number of lysosomes.

The view that epithelioid cells are a rather distinct variety of macrophage has recently been cogently argued by Papadimitriou and Spector (1971), who studied the cells appearing under various circumstances on implanted cellophane. These cells which certainly look quite like the epithelioid cells of granulomata are of bone marrow origin and contain a moderate quantity of granular endoplasmic reticulum and lysosomes. They synthesize RNA—presumably in relation to their ability to synthesize lysosomes; they are poorly phagocytic towards bacteria but can pinocytose small particles and degrade iodinated proteins. They can divide (some 1% take up tritiated thymidine) and when they do their progeny are small round cells which may be able to mature into epithelioid cells. Their development, it is postulated, is dependent on the absence of persistent indigestible material within the cell.

Views on the precursors of the epithelioid cell vary. Epstein *et al.* (1963) who used thymidine labelling in human experimental granulomas suggested that epithelioid cells derived directly from small mononuclear cells. In granulomata induced by the injection of mycobacterial cell wall components on the other hand, Galindo *et al.* (1969) postulated a series of gradations between blast cells, macrophages and epithelioid cells containing numerous large lysosomes.

The structure of macrophages in granulomata may be modified by the persistence within the cell of the causative organism—the brucella or the leprosy bacillus (Karlsbad *et al.*, 1964; Allen *et al.*, 1965). After the phagocytosis of toxic siliceous dusts there may be extensive necrosis of macrophages.

Giant cells develop from macrophages in granulomata (Davis, 1964; Gusek, 1964; Sutton and Weiss, 1965; Sutton, 1967). Both the so-called "tuberculous" and "foreign-body" giant cells probably develop in a similar way. Single macrophages interlock their adjacent processes and the interdigitating cytoplasmic membranes may then disappear. The process might be regarded as the opposite of that involved in the formation of new cytoplasmic membrane in cell division (Fig. 46).

Macrophages with very numerous cytoplasmic processes have been observed in peripheral lymph at various sites including the lymph draining granulomata. There is evidence that there is a continuous cellular traffic through granulomata; lymphocytes and monocytes pass out of the blood; the monocytes presumably mature into macrophages in the granulomata and migrate therefrom into the draining lymph node (Smith *et al.*, 1970a b). At least some granulomata contain capillaries with high endothelial cells similar to those in lymph nodes.

The role of the monocytes in the development of chronic inflammatory lesions has been extensively studied by Spector and his colleagues. These workers initially studied the effects of injection of various proteins into the skin of the rat.

Polymorphs and monocytes migrate out of blood vessels simultaneously, but only the monocytes persist and mature; the migration rate of monocytes was maximal 3–5 h and 8–24 h after the stimulus, i.e. migration was biphasic (Paz and Spector, 1962; Boughton and Spector, 1963).

Spector and Lykke (1966) studied the development of an experimental granuloma using thymidine labelling and autoradiography to follow cells which were undergoing DNA synthesis, and carbon labelling to trace phagocytic cells. It was found that after blood monocytes had emigrated from blood vessels they divided over a period of 12 weeks or more. There was also some division by cells in blood vessel walls. The lesion persisted largely because of this proliferation aided to some extent by further migration of cells. Cells laden with particulate matter did not usually divide. When they did the particulate matter was taken up by young histiocytes. When tritiated thymidine was given before the start of the lesion, epithelioid cells and giant cells were found to be labelled; this was evidence that these cells were of recent origin and probably derived from macrophages. Clusters of small round cells were noted as a characteristic feature of these, as of many, granulomas. Appropriate pulse labelling of these cells with tritiated thymidine showed that they probably originated from larger pale staining cells (blast cells). The authors put forward the hypothesis that these cells form part of a cellular cycle, being themselves derived from macrophages and being capable of maturation into macrophages.

The rate of migration of monocytes and polymorphs into a granuloma was studied by transfusing blood containing labelled cells into the animal (Spector *et al.*, 1967). The rate of emigration of polymorphs, initially high, fell off rapidly, whereas monocytes entered the lesion at a constant rate of 200,000 in 24 h for up to 12 weeks; the entry rate of the two cell types seemed to be independently controlled suggesting the existence of separate factors stimulating migration of the two cell types. After entering the lesion further division of monocytes occurs. In other granulomatous lesions migration of monocytes was almost complete 24 h after the initial stimulus and any subsequent increase in mononuclear cells is attributable largely to cell division (Spector and Coote, 1965). Irradiation of the marrow abolishes the inflammatory reaction which may be restored by marrow cells (Spector and Willoughby, 1968). The same general conclusions were reached from similar thymidine-labelling studies in the mouse by Van Furth and Cohn (1968).

The factors involved in producing chronicity in inflammatory lesions of rat skin have been studied by Spector *et al.* (1968) and reviewed by Spector (1969). After injection of natural proteins and synthetic polymers into rat skin the lesions were studied histologically after carbon and tritiated thymidine labelling. The mononuclear infiltration lasted longer after injection of synthetic compounds, and was clearly related to the molecular size of the polymer. Cell proliferation declines after 3 days unless the lesion is going to become chronic. Chronicity is associated with persistence of the stimulus in the tissues, notably intracellular persistence.

Ryan and Spector (1969, 1970) further studied cell turnover in granulomas induced by various stimuli. They found that granulomas fell into two types. In one, exemplified by the carrageenin lesion, the mature granuloma was largely composed of macrophages laden with carrageenin. The emigration rate and cell division rate was low. The life cycle of macrophages was up to 2 months.

In other forms of granuloma, exemplified by those induced by injection of pertussis, TAB, or paraffin oil, a lower proportion of macrophages contain the irritant and there is a continuous emigration and turnover of cells in the lesion. This is a proliferative lesion. Even here some macrophages live up to 2 months. The authors postulate natural selection of a clone of long-lived cells able to survive ingestion of the irritant.

Low turnover granulomas contain many stable long-lived mature macrophages presumably laden with the causative irritant. High turn-over granulomas, on the other hand, contain many young monocytes. The lesion induced by BCG contains a mixture of cells, including epithelioid cells (Papadimitriou and Spector, 1972). It is likely that the high turnover lesions contain many cells which are readily damaged by endocytosis and that the low turnover lesions contain long surviving cells of high phagocytic ability. It seems that natural selection of long-lived cells may occur in such lesions explaining the tendency of high turnover lesions in time to change into low turnover lesions (Spector, 1969). Apart from the turnover of macrophages in granulomas there is good evidence that in at least some granulomas large numbers of lymphocytes are produced.

Granulomatous reactions are induced by many stimuli; the most important common factor seems to be the persistence of material undegraded in component macrophages. Spector *et al.* (1970) studied the rate of disposal in tissues of injected bacteria labelled with ^{125}I. Breakdown of organisms which did not induce granuloma formation was almost complete within 48 h of injection; a significant fraction of organisms which did induce granuloma formation on the other hand persisted undegraded in the tissues for more than 48 h.

An important granuloma is that induced by silica; the silica particles are ingested by macrophages and find their way into secondary lysosomes. They cause rupture of lysosomal membranes, possibly due to hydrogen bonding of silicic acid to the phospholipid membranes of the lysosome. The lysosomal enzymes are then released into the cell, killing it (Allison *et al.*, 1966; Allison, 1970). The silica is then ingested by other macrophages, only to kill them. Macrophages which have ingested silica release a factor which stimulates fibroblasts to synthesize collagen (Heppleston and Styles, 1967).

In the granuloma induced by asbestos Davis (1963a, b, 1964) demonstrated that when asbestos particles are ingested by macrophages they become coated by ferritin. In this lesion giant cells are prominent, formed by interdigitation of the cytoplasmic processes of adjacent macrophages, but it is doubtful whether the giant cells remain highly phagocytic. Asbestos bodies found in the sputum in asbestosis are formed by ingestion or partial ingestion of asbestos fibres by macrophages, followed by degeneration of the macrophage, leaving a ferritin coated fibre (Holt and Young, 1967; Botham and Holt, 1968).

Where bacteria cause a granuloma they may persist alive within the macrophages for a long time, for instance in tuberculosis or leprosy (Dumont and Sheldon, 1965; Allen *et al.*, 1965). The intracellular survival of tubercle bacilli in cultured macrophages may be associated with a failure of fusion of secondary lysosomes and phagosomes (Armstrong and Hart, 1971). Similarly in macrophages which had ingested histoplasma, some organisms persisted apparently intact and without evidence of fusion of phagosome and lysosome (Dumont and Robert, 1970), and alveolar macrophages from cortisone-treated mice showed failure of fusion of lysosomes with phagosomes containing aspergillus (Merkow, Epstein *et al.*, 1971). The balance between the macrophage and an infecting organism may be affected by a third factor; for instance silica potentiates the growth of the tubercle bacillus in macrophages in tissue culture, possibly by damaging their lysosomes. Conversely chemotherapeutic agents may affect the balance in a similar way, though this is less common. Hart (1968) suggested that some detergents modify growth of tubercle bacilli by being stored in lysosomes. Certainly the antituberculous riminophenazines are stored in macrophages in large amounts (Conalty and Jackson, 1962).

In summary a granuloma may be seen as a device whereby a temporary outpost of the lymphoreticular system is established in the tissues, in which large numbers of mature macrophages are immobilized in the area and may divide and in which considerable numbers of lymphocytes may be pronounced.

The "Immune Macrophage"

It has been suggested that as part of the immune response under certain circumstances specifically sensitized immune macrophages may appear. This field has been reviewed by Nelson (1969) and Stuart (1970). While macrophages play an important part in the development and expression of immunity there is no real evidence that any mysterious entity, the "immune macrophage", exists (see Mackaness and Blanden, 1967). What does happen is that after exposure to an infection which elicits cell-mediated immunity macrophages are induced to mature (e.g. North, 1969a, b, 1970a, b). This maturation may involve both free and fixed macrophages. The mature macrophages contain increased quantities of hydrolytic enzymes and have an increased ability to spread on glass, but their increased function is largely non-specific.

A series of studies on "immune" macrophages has been carried out by Hard (1969, 1970), on peritoneal cells from mice immune to *Corynebacterium ovis*. As compared to normal cells the "immune" cells were larger, showed less evidence of pinocytosis, contained more protein and more of the seven hydrolytic enzymes measured (acid phosphatase, β-glucuronidase, cathepsin D, β-naphthol esterase, β-naphthyl-acetate esterase and aryl sulphatase). "Immune" macrophages consumed less oxygen than normal cells but were twice as active in glycolysis. ATP levels were five times less than in normal macrophages and protein synthesis measured by glycerine uptake, half as much. The "immune" cells contained many more lysosomal granules. All these features are merely the characteristics of full cellular maturity.

The development of cellular immunity to *Listeria monocytogenes* has been studied by North (1969a, b). After a wave of vigorous proliferation of fixed phagocytes lining the liver sinusoids and of resident macrophages in the peritoneal cavity a population of macrophages appears with increased physiological and microbicidal ability. Suppression of the proliferation of Kupffer cells did not inhibit the development of immunity but total body irradiation or a prior pulse of the antimitotic agent vinblastine did, presumably by destroying the precursors of migrant macrophages.

The weight of evidence therefore favours the view that the increased avidity shown by macrophages in immune lesions can be explained either by non-specific maturation of cells, or by the presence of a layer of cytophilic antibody on their surfaces. The true "immune macrophage" would be a cell which had an ability to phagocytose and destroy one specific organism for reasons other than the presence of antibody absorbed on its surface. There is not as yet good evidence that such a cell exists.

The Uptake and Processing of Antigen

Much work has been done on the uptake of antigens by macrophages; only a limited account will be given here. The field is fully reviewed, e.g. by Humphrey (1969) and Nelson (1969). It should first of all be emphasized that macrophages are essential only in some immune responses. For instance Mandel *et al.* (1969) have shown that lymphoid cells can react directly with some antigens, characteristically those presenting in finely divided form like ferritin. In some situations uptake of antigen may actually depress the immune response (Perkins and Makinodan, 1965).

Antigenic substances are of course taken up by macrophages non-specifically. Han *et al.* (1970) observed that isologous ferritin was taken up by lymph node macrophages in small amounts by micropinocytosis whereas heterologous ferritin was taken up by the same mechanism in much larger amounts; presumably the latter process involves specific recognition by the macrophage. Nossall *et al.* (1968a, b) suggested that the bacterial protein flagellin might enter macrophages by pinocytosis, micropinocytosis or direct penetration of the membrane; the latter is somewhat dubious. Two antigens may be taken up without preference by

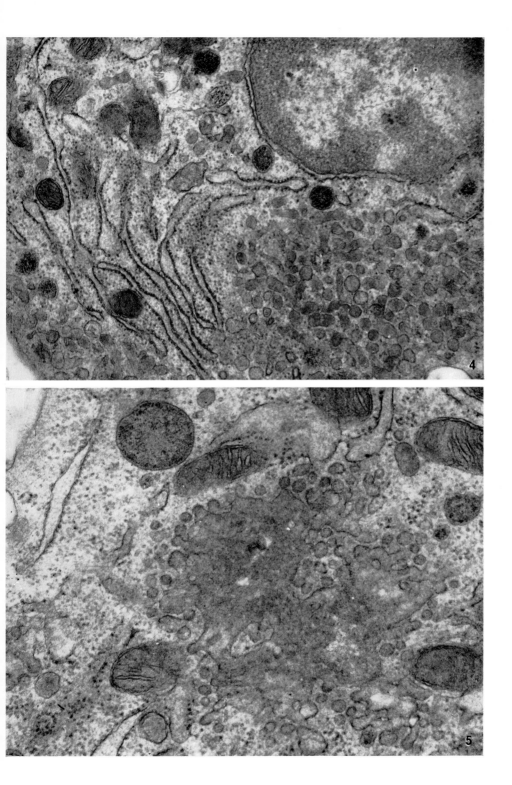

Figure 6. Peritoneal macrophage; acid phosphatase preparation showing deposit in lysosomes. × 25,000.

Figure 7. Cell coat of peritoneal macrophage with deep invaginations on the surface crossed by fine strands of coat substance. The coat substance is in globular aggregates in places and is adherent to the outer layer of the unit membrane. × 85,000.

Figure 8. Lysosome from stimulated mouse peritoneum showing unit membrane at periphery, and an electron lucent area deep to the membrane. The core is composed of a granular electron dense substance in which ferritin is not evident (from through focus series). × 123,000

Figure 9. Detail of similar lysosome showing paracrystalline array of dense granules (from a through focus series). × 159,000

Figure 10. Peritoneal macrophage (mouse) stimulated by incubating *in vitro* with a lipid emulsion. The cell surface is highly irregular showing numerous cytoplasmic processes. × 13,000.

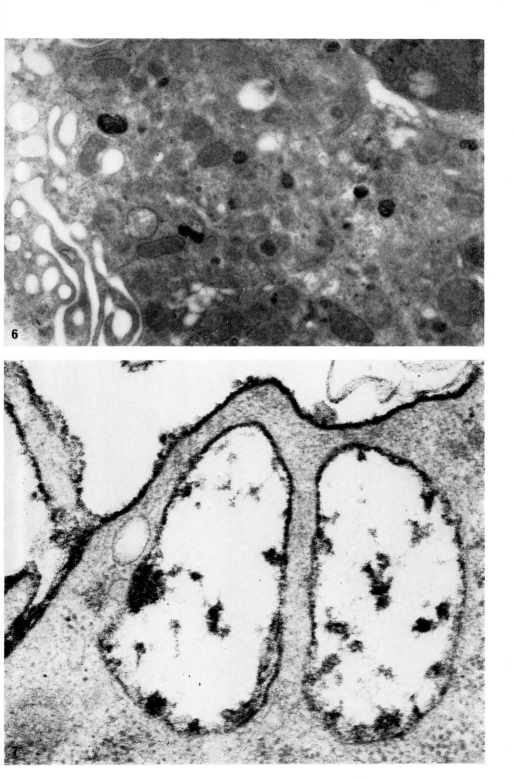

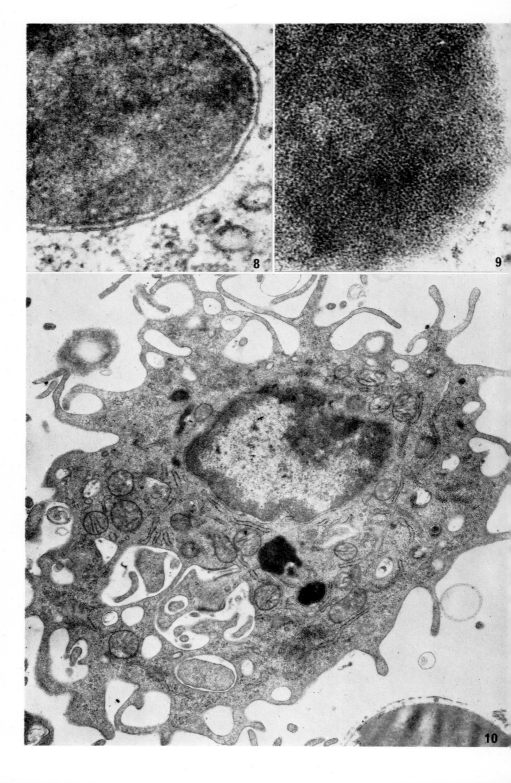

8

9

10

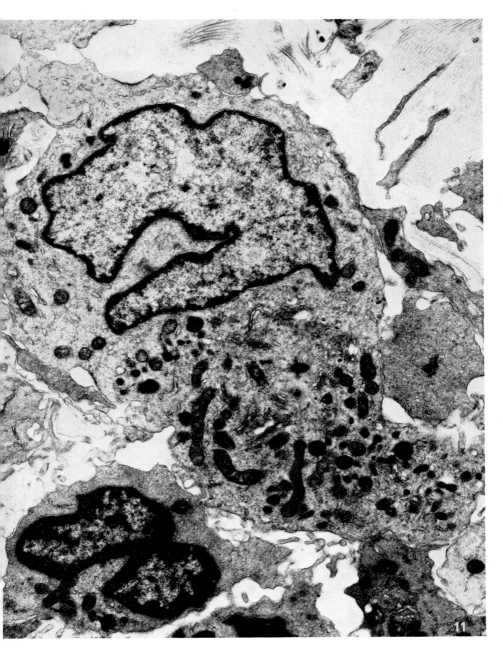

Figure 11. Histiocyte (human) from subcutaneous tissue adjacent to neoplasm. The cytoplasm contains rather scanty membranous structures and a few small lysosomes. × 11,000.

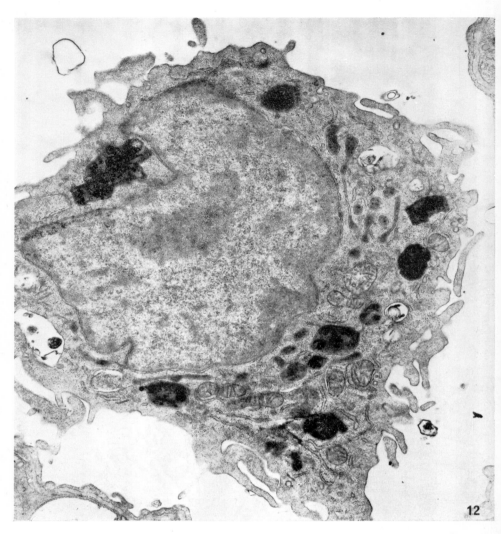

Figure 12. Alveolar macrophage (mouse). Numerous irregular lysosomes are present, some of which contain carbon derived from the atmosphere. × 14,000.

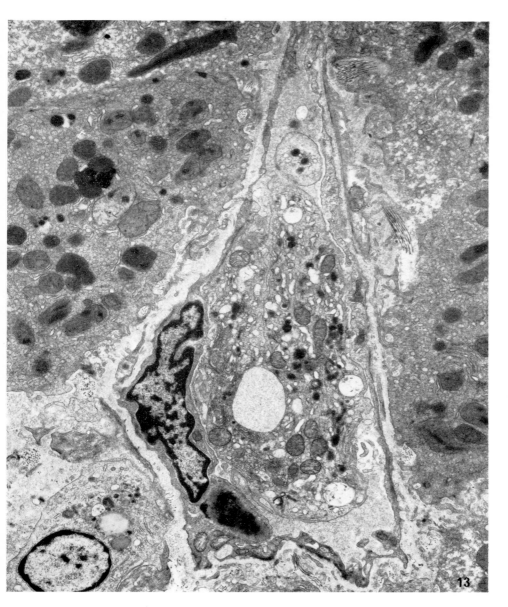

Figure 13. Liver – Kupffer cell (human). The cytoplasm of the Kupffer cell lies apparently free in the sinusoid. It contains several large vacuoles and numerous small lysosomes. The wall of the vessel is made up at this point of very thin endothelium. Outside the vessel are hepatic epithelial cells and a paravascular macrophage. × 8,000.

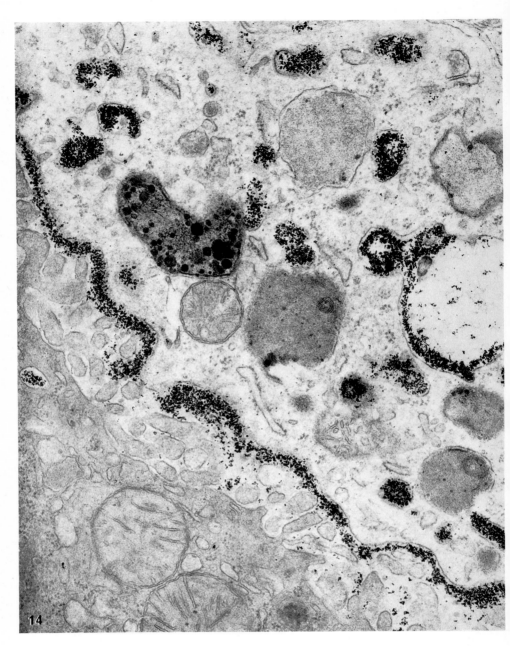

Figure 14. Kupffer cell cytoplasm (mouse). This animal had received an intravenous dose of thorotrast one hour before sacrifice. Thorotrast is adherent to the Kupffer cell but not to an adjacent hepatic epithelial cell: thorotrast is also present in vacuoles and vesicles within the Kupffer cell. Some of the secondary lysosomes are of markedly heterogeneous structure. × 33,000.

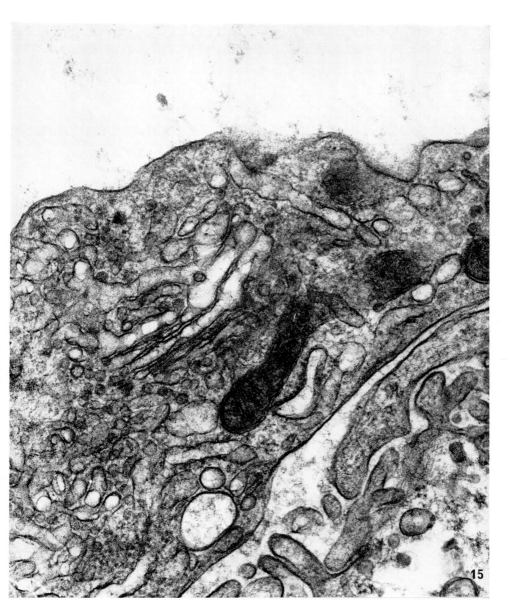

Figure 15. Kupffer cell (mouse) showing the intracytoplasmic tubular channels characteristic of these cells. An incomplete "fuzzy coat" lies on the luminal surface of the cell membrane. × 49,000.

Figure 16. Splenic sinusoid (human). A red blood cell and a lymphocyte are passing through the wall of the sinusoid at different points. The cytoplasm of the sinus endothelial cells contains numerous dense areas. A basement membrane of variable thickness lies deep to the endothelial cells. × 10,000.

Figure 17. Splenic sinusoid (human). At higher magnification these dense areas are formed by aggregation of fine microfibrils forming a feltwork. These microfibrils appear to branch (arrows). × 66,000.

Figure 18. Splenic macrophage (human). The cytoplasm contains a large inclusion recognizably composed of an ingested cell. × 11,000.

Figure 19. Splenic macrophage (human). The detail of an inclusion bound by a unit membrane and containing a granular substructure and some small membranous fragments. This probably represents a degenerate phagocytosed RBC. × 32,000.

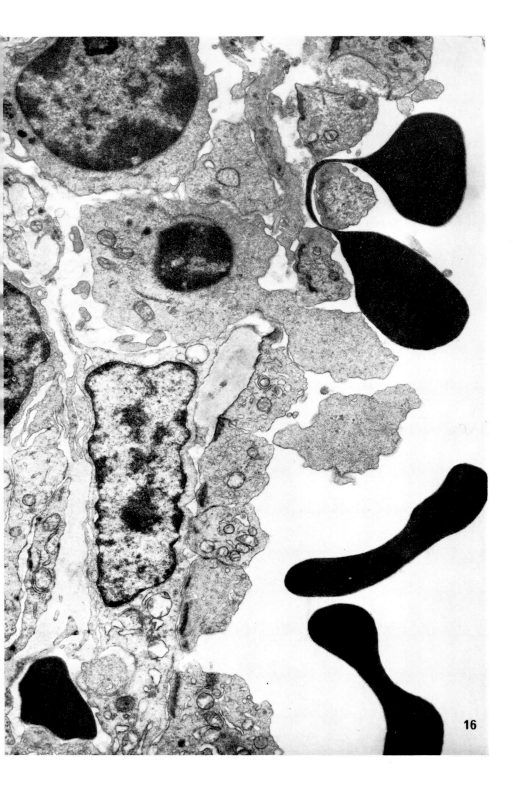

16

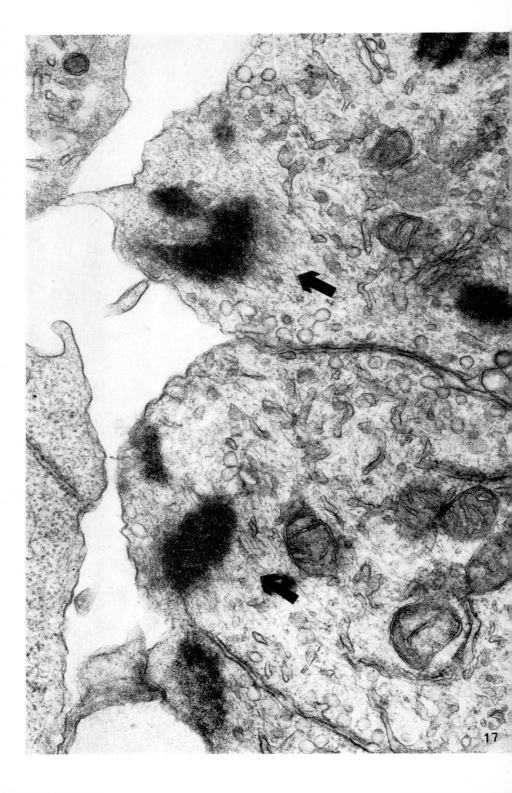

17

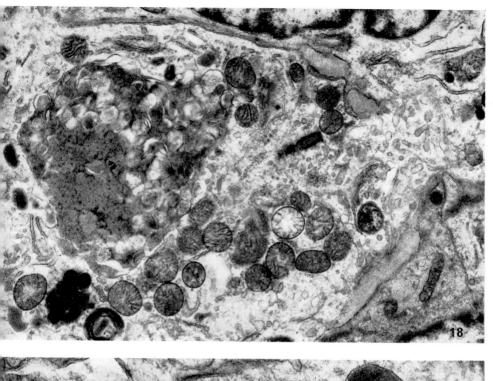

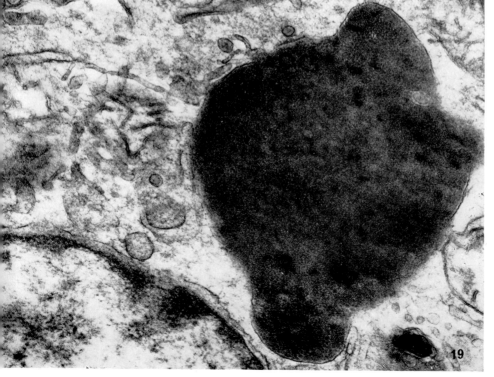

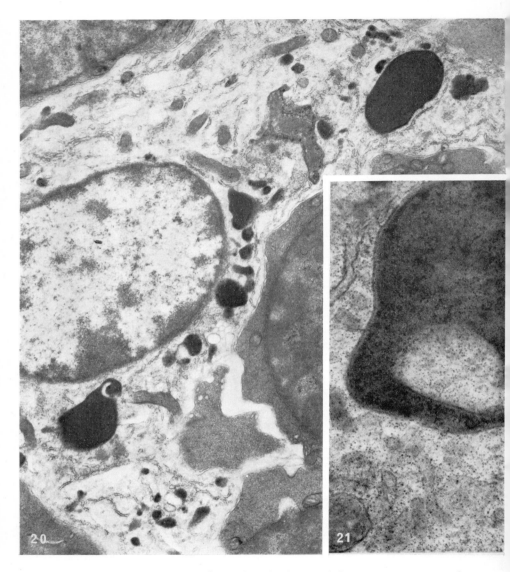

Figure 20. Marrow macrophage (monkey) containing numerous secondary lysosomes of highly variable size and shape. × 11,000.

Figure 21. Detail of inclusion from marrow macrophage. Large amounts of ferritin are found both within lysosomes and free in the cytoplasm. × 74,000.

Figure 22. Lymph node, subcapsular sinus (mouse). The capsule is formed of several layers of fibroblasts with collagen in between. The sinus is lined on its superficial surface by flattened endothelial cells and on its deep surface partly by similar cells and partly by macrophages. Macrophages lie across the lumen of the sinus sometimes apparently free, sometimes adherent to one another. × 3,000.

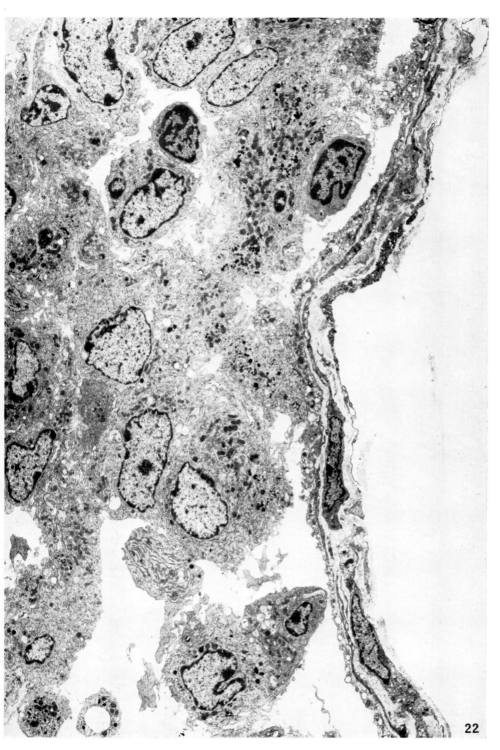

22

E

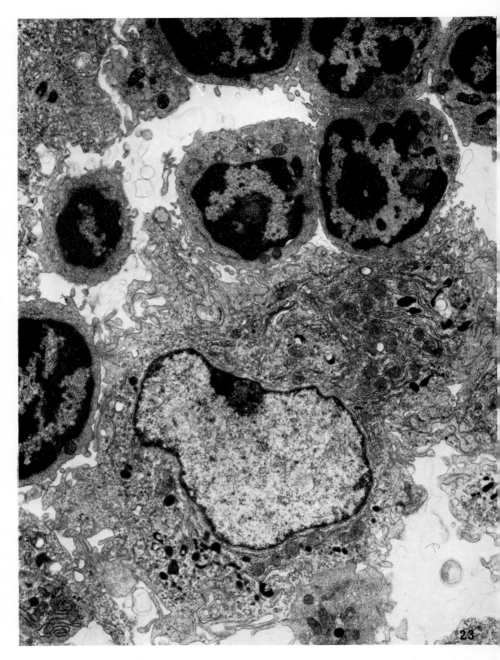

Figure 23. An interstitial macrophage from a lymph node (mouse). There is well developed granular endoplasmic reticulum, and a moderate number of small lysosomes. The surface shows numerous cytoplasmic flaps. The cell lies in close relationship with adjacent lymphocytes. × 9,300.

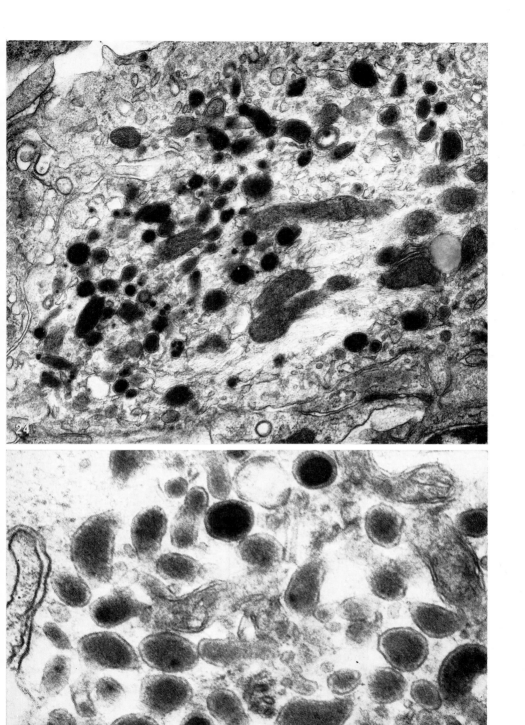

Figure 24. Cytoplasm of interstitial macrophage (mouse lymph node). Numerous dense bodies contain cores of varying electron density. The cell is attached to an adjacent macrophage by a desmosome. × 25,000.

Figure 25. Group of lysosomal dense bodies from similar cell. Each is bounded by a unit membrane deep to which is a pale rim. The core contains numerous fine granules and is sometimes highly electron dense. × 62,000.

Figure 26. The edge of a macrophage from a mouse popliteal lymph node showing numerous microfibrils, 6 nm in diameter, criss-crossing and sometimes apparently branching. × 71,000.

Figure 27. Macrophages from popliteal lymph node showing an aggregate of microtubules with microfibrils lying at the edge of the aggregate. × 31,000.

Figure 28. Interstitial reticulum cell (rat popliteal lymph node). The cell is in mitosis. The rat had received 5 million tumour cells into the footpad 24 h before, and showed very early metastasis. × 7000.

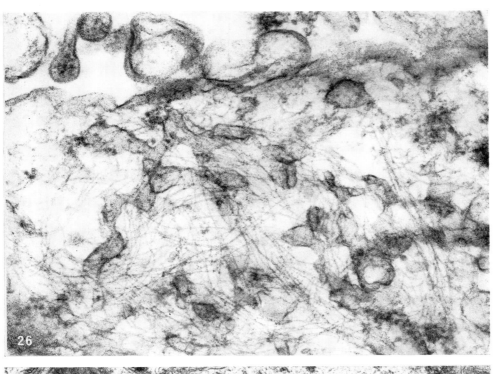

26

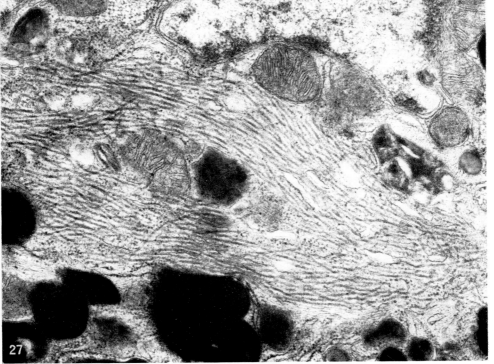

27

Figure 29. Interstitial reticulum cell (mouse popliteal lymph node). Several autoradiographic grains overlie the nucleus. The mouse had received a priming dose of antigen, followed by a second dose into the footpad. ³H-thymidine was given 1 h before killing. Autoradiograph × 9000.

Figure 30. Part of macrophage from subarachnoid space of newborn mouse (choroid plexus region). Such cells often have long cytoplasmic flaps and large vacuoles and resemble Hofbauer cells. × 17,000.

Figure 31. Small microglial cell (newborn mouse cerebral cortex). The appearance is that of a small immature macrophage with some granular endoplasmic recitulum, small cytoplasmic dense bodies, lipid vacuoles and larger dense bodies probably secondary lysosomes. × 11,000

Figure 32. Detail of microglial cell showing small homogeneous and large heterogeneous dense bodies. × 18,000

Figure 33. Hofbauer cell from human placenta. Such cells characteristically have long processes with large vacuole like invaginations. Similar large vesicles occur within the cell. × 12,000

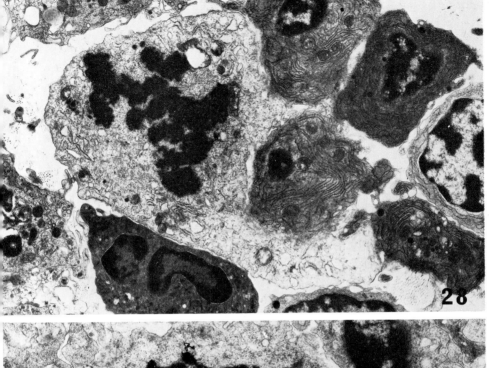

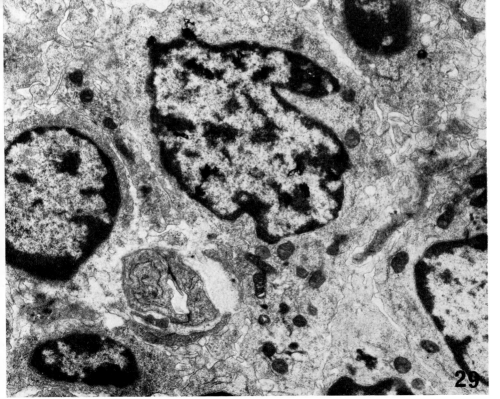

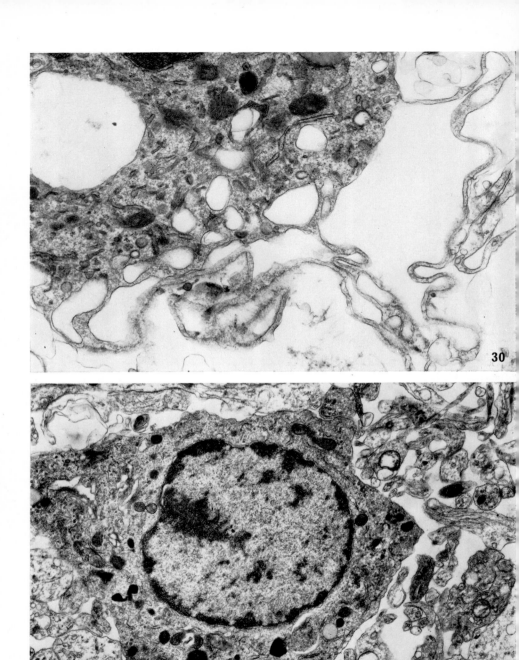

30

31

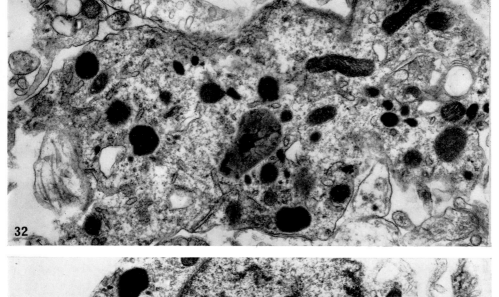

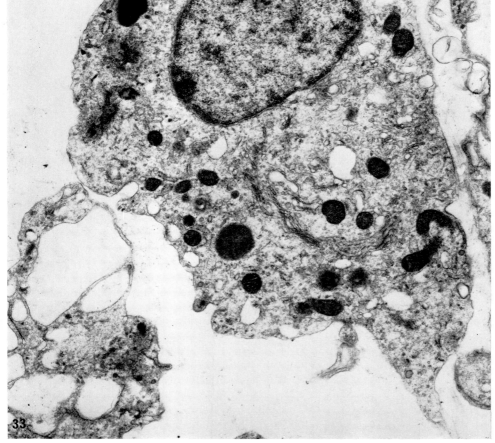

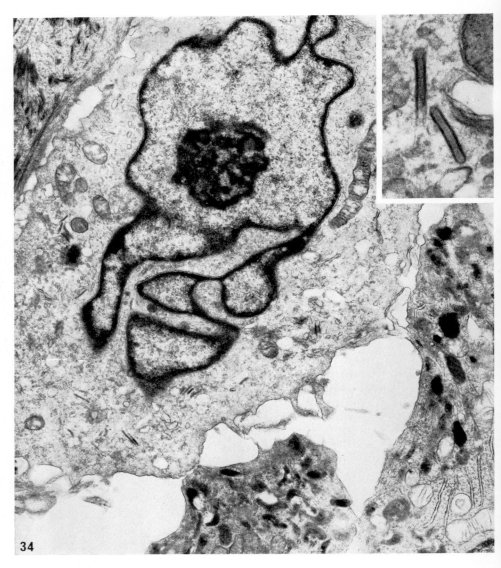

Figure 34. Langerhans cell from human epidermis. The cell has in general rather unspecialized cytoplasmic organization but contains small rod-shaped structures. These (inset) are bounded by a unit membrane and have an electron dense core which shows faint periodic banding. × 13,000.

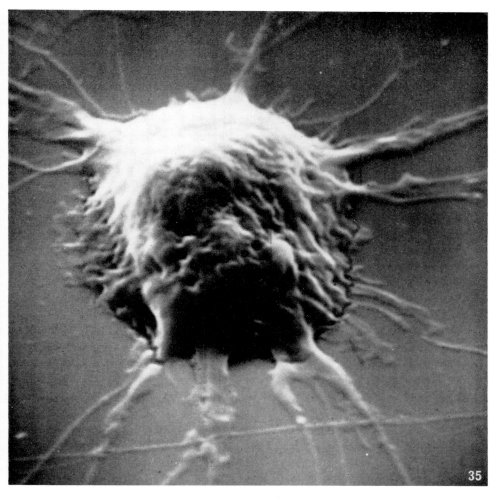

35

Figure 35. Mouse peritoneal macrophage which has been allowed to settle on glass for 8 hours. It has extruded fine probe-like cytoplasmic processes in all directions and also wide flap-like processes. The process running transversely across the bottom of the picture derives from another macrophage. The depressions on the upper surface are of the right size to be the structures usually called vacuoles when cut in cross section in a transmission micrograph. Scanning EM. × 10,000.

Figure 36. Blood monocyte. The nucleus is deeply indented and there are numerous juxtanuclear microfibrils. Small cytoplasmic processes at the edge of the cell enclose small invaginations. The cytoplasm contains a few small lysosomes. × 13,000.

Figure 37. A group of mononuclear cells adherent to a lipid globule (mouse peritoneal cells). The cytoplasm of the phagocytes is spread out over the surface of the globule. × 3,000.

Figure 38. Detail of the above showing the very close apposition between the phagocyte and the lipid globule. × 12,000.

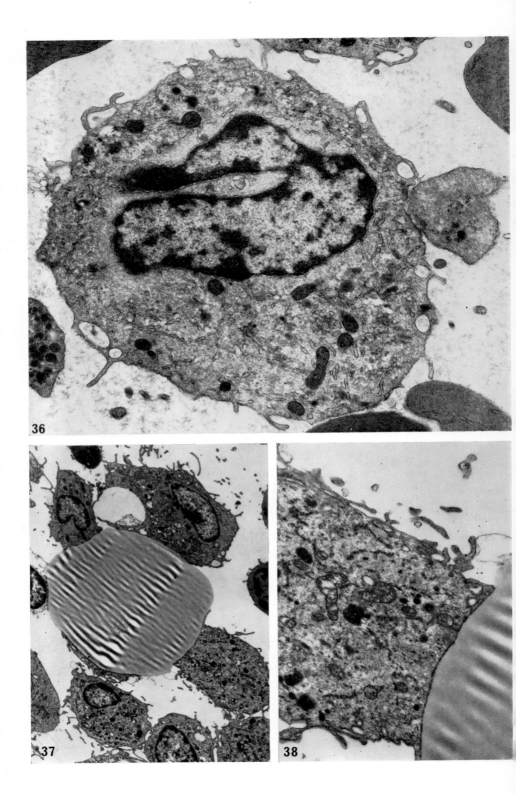

36

37   38

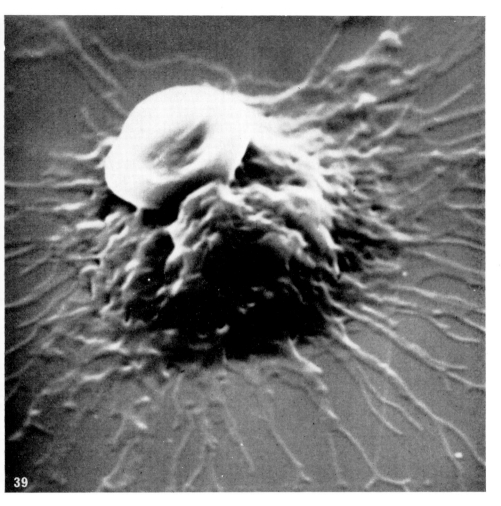

Figure 39. Mouse peritoneal macrophage settled on glass (as Fig. 35) phagocytosing a red blood cell. Note the flap of cytoplasm pushing up the lower side
of the red blood corpuscle. Scanning EM. × 10,000.

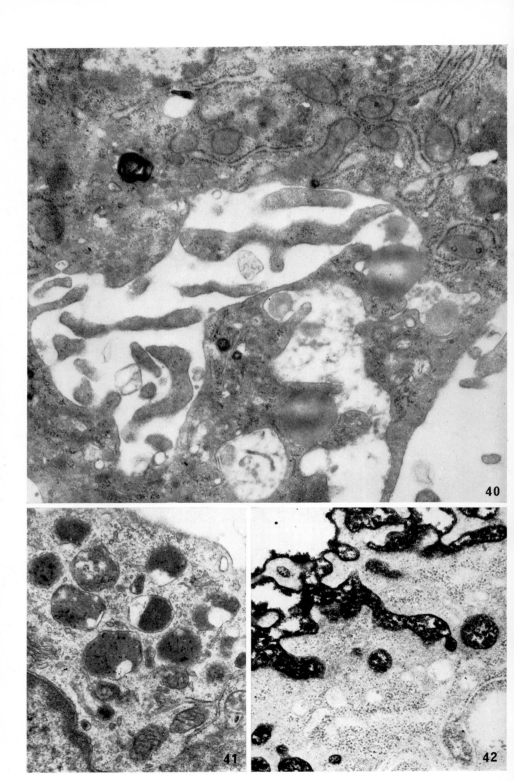

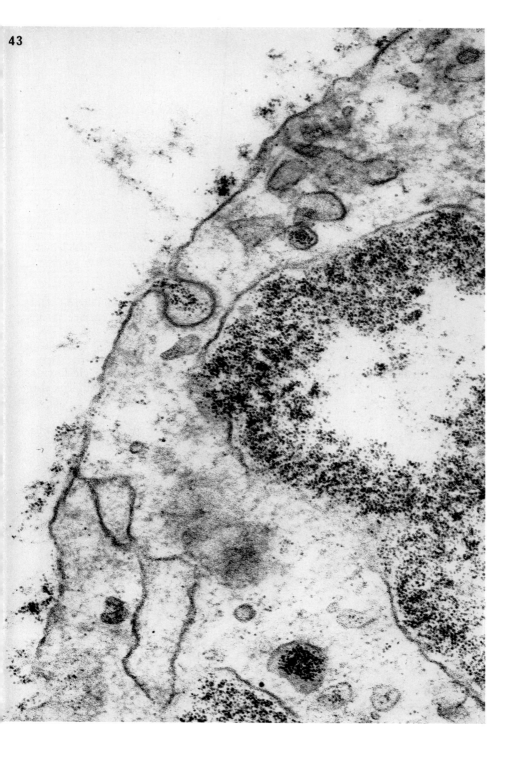

Figure 40. Mouse peritoneal macrophage phagocytosing lipid globules which are held in a deep invagination of the cell surface. × 25,000.

Figure 41. Mouse peritoneal macrophage from an animal given colloidal gold intraperitoneally after prior stimulation with a lipid emulsion. Particles are present in the large but not the small lysosomes. The former are therefore clearly secondary lysosomes. × 20,000.

Figure 42. Pinocytosis induced by incubation of mouse peritoneal macrophages in a solution containing ferritin. Deep channels invaginate the surface of the cell. The cell coat is stained with ruthenium red. × 20,000.

Figure 43. Sinusoidal macrophage from mouse popliteal node showing ingestion of heterologous ferritin by micropinocytosis in a coated vesicle. The ferritin is held in little packets on the surface of the cell. Part of a large vacuole is also visible. × 100,000.

Figure 44. Granuloma macrophage from human sarcoidosis. The pseudopodia of adjacent cells are pressed against one another and sometimes interdigitate. The cell contains numerous small fairly homogeneous lysosomes. Endoplasmic reticulum is less prominent in this profile than in others. × 10,000.

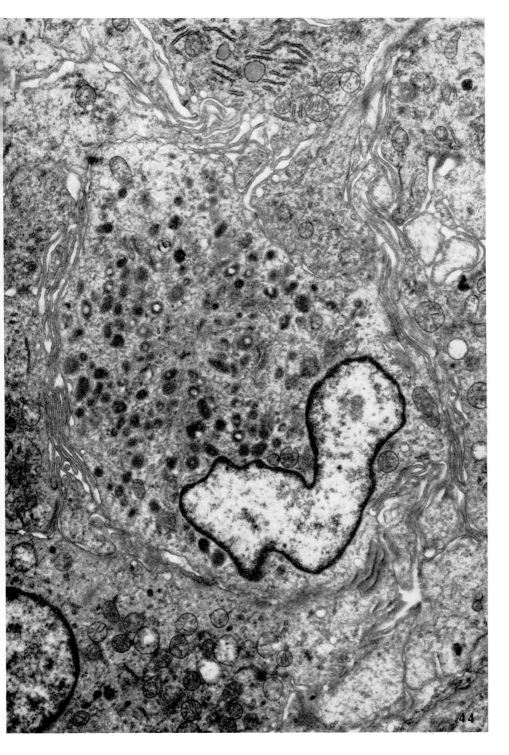

44

F

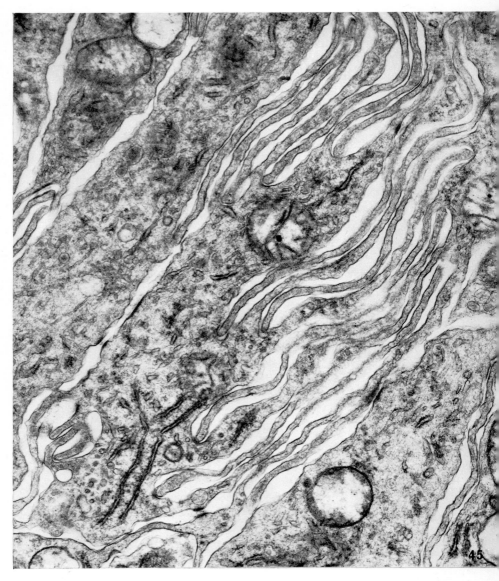

Figure 45. Detail of interdigitating cell process from the above. Adjacent cells are held together by poorly formed desmosomes. × 22,000.

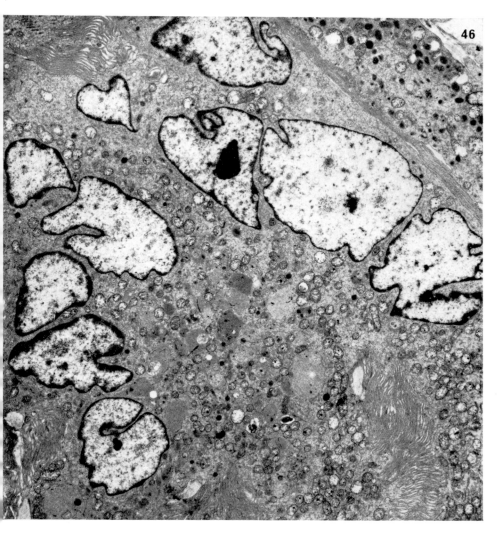

Figure 46. Giant multinucleate cell from the above. There is a moderate number of large rather electron lucent inclusions and large arrays of inter-digitating stacked membranes. × 5,000.

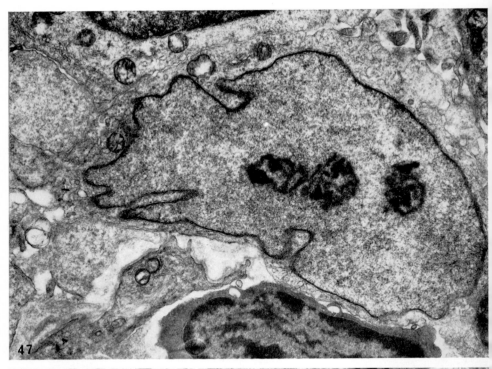

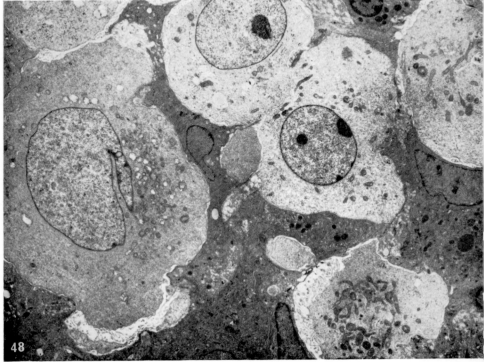

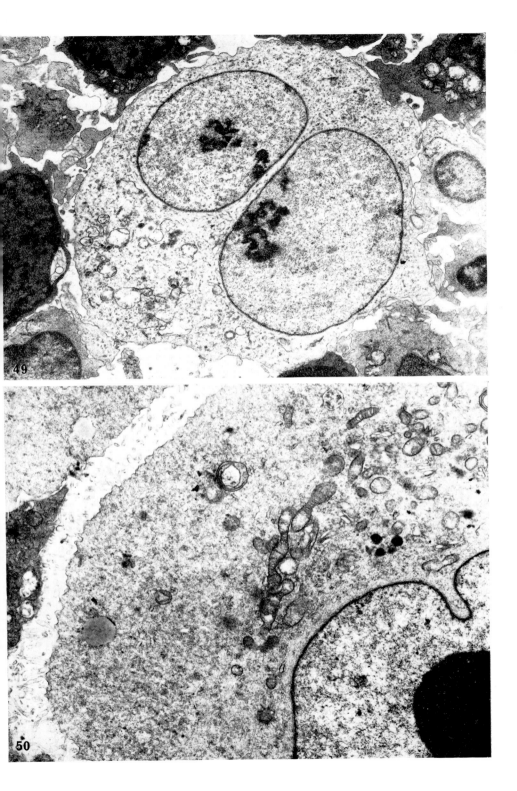

49

50

Figure 47. A relatively small elongated cell with elongated and indented nucleus from a normal human lymph node; the nucleolus is prominent. This would be best described as a small reticulum cell. From a normal human lymph node. × 10,000.

Figure 48. Survey micrograph of a lymph node from a patient with Hodgkin's disease, showing large abnormal reticulum cells with electron lucent cytoplasm. The cells have numerous fine cytoplasmic processes. × 3,000.

Figure 49. Binucleate reticulum cell from lymph node from a patient with Hodgkin's disease. The nuclei contain prominent nucleoli. The cytoplasm shows several small strands of endoplasmic reticulum and a moderate number of scattered free RNP particles. The mitochondria, as often in these cells, show degenerative changes. × 11,000.

Figure 50. Detail of abnormal reticulum cell from lymph node from patient with Hodgkin's disease. There are numerous small cytoplasmic processes, a cluster of mitochondria near the cell centre, small lysosomes and a small fat droplet. The nucleolus is prominent. × 10,000.

Figure 51. Great alveolar cell from mouse lung. A mass of cytoplasm protrudes into the lumen of the alveolus (top). The cytoplasm contains numerous electron-dense osmiophilic myelin bodies, and several large mitochondria. × 21,000.

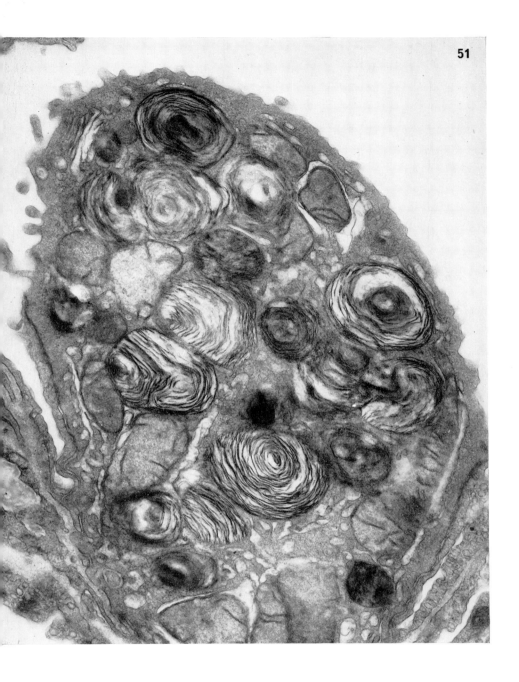

Figure 52. Mesothelial cells from mouse omentum. Thin flattened leaflets of cytoplasm abut at a desmosome. The cells have thin finger-like processes and numerous micropinocytic vesicles. × 13,000; inset × 20,000.

Figure 53. Sertoli cell from rat testis. The flattened nucleus of the cell lies against the capsule of the seminiferous tubule; the cell has a prominent Golgi apparatus and a cluster of lysosomes. × 7,000.

Figure 54. Epithelial reticular cell from mouse thymus. The cytoplasm contains microfibrillar aggregates and vacuoles containing microvilli. × 22,000.

Figure 55. A multinucleate osteoclast from metaphysis of neonatal rat femur. Note the brush border (arrow) lying adjacent to a trabecula of bone. × 10,000.

Figure 56. Detail of brush border. Fine spicules of calcium salts lie between cytoplasmic processes from the osteoclast. Bone matrix arrowed. × 20,000.

Figure 57. Sinus macrophage (rat popliteal lymph node). The cell is in mitosis. The rat had received 5 million tumour cells into the footpad 24 h before, and showed very early metastasis in the popliteal node. × 9000.

Figure 58. Neoplastic cell (bottom left) and macrophage from rat transplantable tumour; the animal had previously been immunized with formalized tumour cells. A fine process of macrophage cytoplasm is closely apposed to the tumour cell. × 9000.

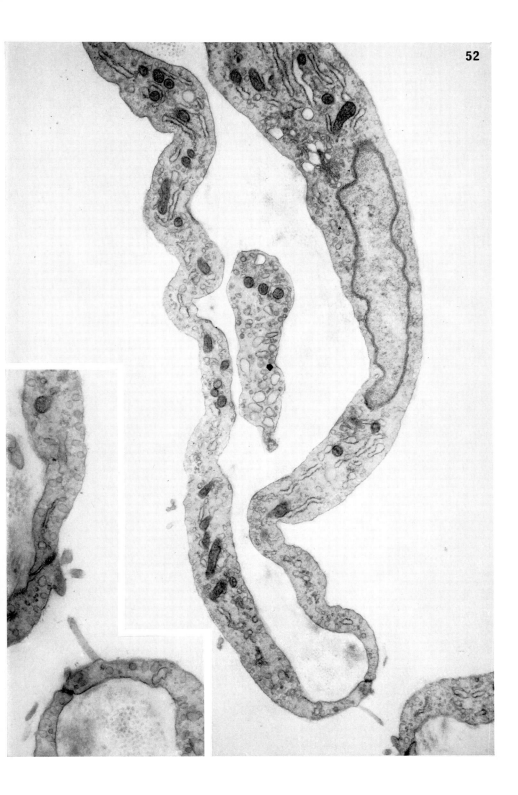

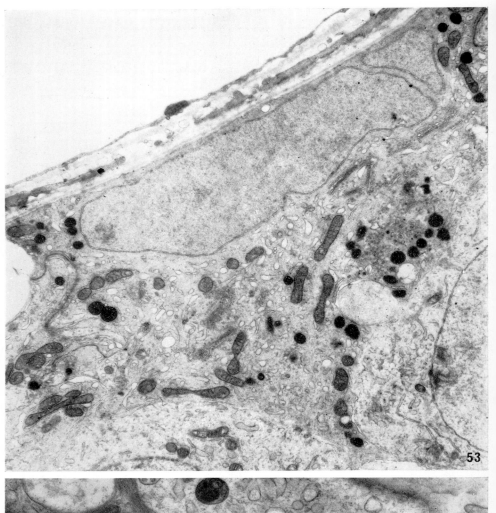

52

53

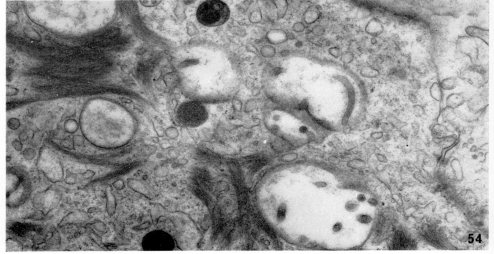

54

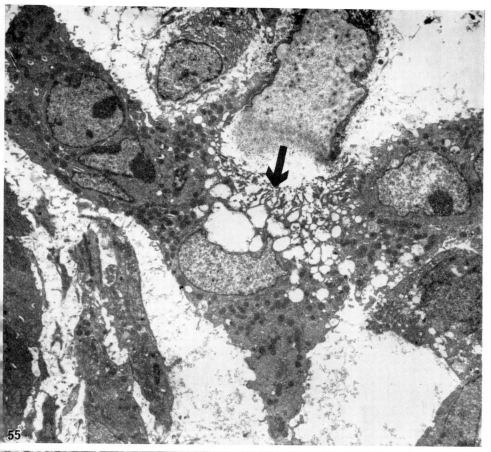

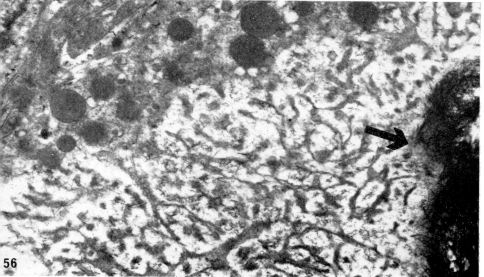

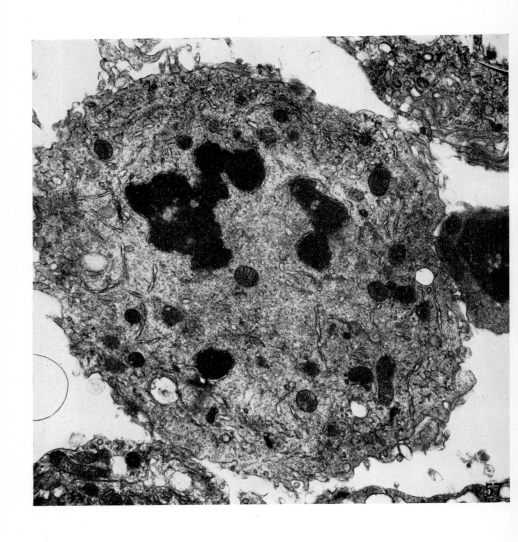

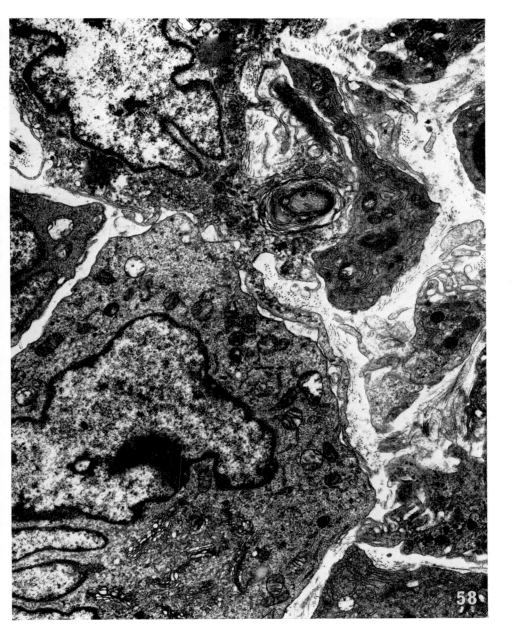

A quite distinct set of observations relates to the interaction between antigens and dendritic macrophages. After injection of various antigens into sensitized animals, antigen is retained on dendritic cells in germinal centres in lymphoid tissue (White, 1963; Nossall *et al.*, 1964; McDevitt *et al.*, 1966; Humphrey *et al.*, 1967). Such cells may degenerate on contact with antigen (Hanna and Szakal, 1968). It appears likely that antigen binds to the surface of dendritic cells, because they carry a superficial layer of adsorbed antibody. The function of this adsorption on to dendritic macrophages is not certain, but it seems possible that the dendritic cell serves as a framework on which lymphocytes can collect and interact with antigen.

There is however conflicting evidence on the significance of the role of dendritic cells. For instance Cohen *et al.* (1966) have shown that non-antigenic particulate materials may lodge in lymphoid follicles in sites which strongly suggest localization on dendritic cells. Straus (1970a, b) studied the response to the antigen horse-radish peroxidase and showed that both antigen and antibody could be present in lymphoblasts and plasma cells, contrary to the findings of Buyukozer *et al.* (1965).

A common method of inducing a more active immune response is by injecting the antigen in a mixture of paraffin oil and killed tubercle bacilli, Freund's adjuvant. Lind (1968) has studied the draining lymph nodes after injection of radioactive flagellin in Freund's adjuvant and has noted that the radioactive label persists around globules of oil in the lymph node. It is possible that these act as depots of antigen, and the oil-water interfaces act as surfaces where antigen and lymphocyte may interact. This is analogous to the postulated function of the dendritic macrophage. Unanue, Askonas and Allison (1969) explored the adjuvant function of the macrophage, using *Bacillus pertussis* as antigen and beryllium sulphate as adjuvant. It was found that macrophages containing both *B. pertussis* and haemocyanin elicited higher antibody levels against haemocyanin than macrophages containing haemocyanin. The adjuvant worked only when taken up by macrophages, but antigen and adjuvant did not need to be in the same macrophage. The catabolism and retention of ^{131}I labelled haemocyanin was not affected by the administration of adjuvant.

A major criticism of much of this work done on the function of macrophages in the immune response is that many of the experiments are highly artificial and use obscure or unnatural antigens given in a way not related to natural disease.

Macrophages have been shown to have some importance in the

maturation of the normal lymphoreticular system. The transplantation of adult macrophages into newborn mice leads to an enhanced immunological response to sheep red blood cells. This suggests that antigen processing is not fully developed in young mice (Argyris, 1968).

Anti-macrophage Serum

It is of some interest that macrophages themselves may be used as antigens in the experimental production of an anti-macrophage serum (AMS). While there are early reports in the literature of sera which have toxic effects on macrophages, serious interest in the subject is recent and follows on extensive work on antilymphocytic serum. Cayeux *et al.* (1966) raised an antiserum in rabbits against mouse macrophages by repeated injections of peritoneal macrophages. The injection of this into mice has little effect. When however the mice received both antimacrophage serum and a haemolytic streptococcus they developed arthritis and cardiopathy, a syndrome rather similar to human rheumatic fever. The mechanism of this is hard to understand because cocci are normally phagocytosed by neutrophil polymorphs. AMS has been clearly shown to inhibit phagocytosis by macrophages (Unanue, 1968; Panijel and Cayeux, 1968; Despont and Cruchaud, 1969; Jennings and Hughes, 1969) and to inhibit antibody formation (Despont and Cruchaud, 1969). It inhibits the primary response to bacteriophage in mice and if given at an appropriate time may accelerate experimental yellow fever. It may actually kill macrophages and can produce histologically visible damage to the walls of splenic sinusoids, despite the fact that the cells lining these sinusoids are not true macrophages.

Cell Killing and the Defence Against Neoplasia

It is well established that the most significant factor in the rejection of a skin graft is killing of the cells of the graft by host cells. The ultrastructure of this has been studied by Wiener *et al.* (1963). It is clear that a very close cytoplasmic contact is established between host mononuclear cells and the cells of the graft but not whether the mononuclear cells act directly on the graft. Nor is it established whether these mononuclear cells are in fact of macrophage lineage.

The administration of silica to animals receiving skin grafts produces widespread destruction of macrophages and prolongs the life of the grafts, suggesting that the effector (killer) cells may be macrophages, perhaps coated with cytophilic antibody (Pearsall and Weiser, 1968a, b).

There is some evidence too, that normal peritoneal macrophages may produce cytotoxic substances. Pincus (1967) showed that when the purified protein derivative of tubercle bacilli is incubated *in vitro* with peritoneal macrophages something appears in the cell free medium which is highly toxic in an immunologically non-specific way to skin and cornea. This cytotoxic factor is probably a phospholipid which acts on cell membranes (Pincus *et al.*, 1971).

The immune response against neoplasms is better seen in experimental neoplasia than in man (reviewed by Alexander, 1968) but is of significance in some human tumours, e.g. melanoma (Lewis *et al.*, 1969). The macrophage plays at least some part in this response. The interaction between macrophages and tumour cells can be studied in the lymph nodes draining tumours or in the tumours themselves. It is well known that in the lymph nodes draining human cancers there may appear in the sinusoids numerous large macrophage-like cells, an appearance known as sinus hyperplasia or sinus histiocytosis. It is not certain where these come from, whether they derive from cells in peripheral lymph or have differentiated from endothelial cells. There is some evidence that prognosis is better in patients whose lymph nodes show marked sinus hyperplasia but none as to the possible mechanisms behind this (Black *et al.*, 1955, 1956).

An experimental counterpart of this effect is provided by the work of Carter and Gershon (1966, 1967) and Gershon and Carter (1967a, b). These workers studied two homotransplantable lymphomas in the hamster, one of which metastasized rapidly, the other of which did not. In the draining lymph nodes of the latter there was a marked sinus hyperplasia and some evidence that the hyperplastic sinus macrophages ingested the neoplastic cells, possibly with a considerable degree of specificity. In the non-metastasizing lesion the macrophages present are mature stimulated cells while in the metastasizing lesion they are immature (Birbeck and Carter, 1972).

A wide variety of lymphoreticular cells can be found in human neoplasms, including macrophages, reticulum cells and cells morphologically similar to dendritic reticular cells; macrophages may be seen in mitosis. There is no ultrastructural evidence that any of these cells are toxic to neoplastic cells possibly because of inhibition by blocking antibody (Underwood and Carr, 1972).

Journey and Amos (1962) described the interaction between macrophages and tumour cells in the peritoneum. The macrophages wrapped processes round the neoplastic cells, rapidly ingesting and digesting them; there was apparent breakdown of the intervening cell membranes with

G

possible cytoplasmic fusion between the two cell types. Bennett *et al.* (1964) showed that sensitized macrophages in tissue culture could ingest and kill tumour cells. Similarly Weiser and his colleagues (Granger and Weiser, 1964; Chambers and Weiser, 1969, 1971, 1972) demonstrated that *in vitro* and in the peritoneal cavity macrophages become closely apposed to tumour cells, the cytoplasmic processes of the two cell types interdigitated, and then the macrophages ingested the tumour cells, either whole or in fragments. Stimulated mature macrophages are more effective at inhibiting tumour cell growth in the peritoneal cavity than less mature macrophages (Ito and Miura, 1966). When peritoneal macrophages from immunized animals react *in vitro*, the macrophages stick to the tumour cells in a similar manner to that described above (Lejeune and Evans, 1972). While in some experimental situations the lymphocytes may be the actual effector cell that kills the tumour cells (Gershon and Carter, 1970) a more attractive general explanation of the relation between lymphocytes and macrophage is that the former produces a substance which sticks to the latter, "arming it", or making it cytotoxic (Evans and Alexander, 1970). Possible mechanisms whereby macrophages may kill tumour cells include the presence on the macrophage surface of a cytotoxic substance, possibly lymphocyte derived, the release of cytotoxic factors by macrophages, phagocytosis of whole tumour cells followed by lysosomal digestion, and the focal attachment of the macrophage to specific local surface areas on the tumour cell, followed by the protrusion of macrophage processes which pinch off portions of the tumour cell.

However, these findings, *in vitro* or in the serosal cavity, do not necessarily relate to the situation in solid neoplasms. Fisher and Fisher (1972) found no evidence of significant relationships between lymphoreticular and neoplastic cells. Hard and Butler (1971) found that in a renal tumour induced by dimethylnitrosamine the initial infiltrate of macrophages was followed later by lymphocytes and plasma cells; the lymphoreticular reaction diminished later on, possibly because it was defeated. Carr *et al.* (1973) have studied the lymphoreticular reaction in a transplantable rat tumour. Numerous macrophages were present insinuating long processes between and phagocytosing, apparently viable, tumour cells (Fig. 58). Lymphocytes lay adjacent in a situation which would have allowed them to "arm" the macrophages. The ultrastructural evidence therefore strongly favours the view that macrophages actively ingest and destroy tumour cells in solid neoplasms. The cellular mechanisms involved require much further investigation.

Chapter Eight

SECRETION BY MACROPHAGES

The release of material by macrophages might involve the egestion of substantially unaltered ingested material, the egestion of an altered residue of ingested material, the release of cytoplasmic material by cellular disintegration or the release of a specifically synthesized cellular product whether by excretion or by partial cellular disintegration; only the last of these possibilities is true secretion and its existence could be proved only by ultrastructural studies. There has not in fact been ultrastructural proof of true secretion by macrophages. There is indeed only scanty ultrastructural evidence for any form of egestion; for instance Sutton and Weiss (1965) illustrated some coated vesicles at the edge of macrophages in culture and postulated that they were passing material out of the cell. Curran and Clark (1964) described the situation where macrophages were attempting to phagocytose a large mass of material; the fact that lysis of the extracellular material can be demonstrated is evidence of secretion of some sort. There is on the other hand considerable functional evidence that macrophages can produce substances of various types, though it is not quite certain whether true secretion is involved.

Anti-bacterial Substances

The production of an antibacterial substance by macrophages *in vitro* was demonstrated by Gershon and Olitski (1965). These workers grew mouse peritoneal cells in the presence and absence of *Salmonella typhi*. On examination of the supernatant they found a group of basic proteins which killed bacteria *in vitro*. The infected culture was a richer source of the antibacterial substance than the non-infected culture. On electrophoresis four distinct substances were obtained of varying bactericidal potency and varying lability to acids, trypsin and heat. This complex of substances was

93

described as monocytin. The possibility has not been eliminated that the substances in question are all merely degradation products of degenerate macrophages.

The antibacterial substance lysozyme was first demonstrated in peritoneal macrophages by Barnes (1941). It is a fairly small basic protein with a high arginine content. There have been several similar demonstrations since, for instance by Myrvik *et al.* (1961), in alveolar macrophages and by Briggs *et al.* (1966), who showed the enzyme to be present in monocytes but not in bone marrow RE cells. Brumfitt and Glynn (1960) cultured *Micrococcus lysodeikticus* with macrophages and polymorphs; organisms which *in vitro* were resistant to lysozyme were not digested by the phagocytes while organisms which were sensitive *in vitro* were digested by phagocytes. The implication is that lysozyme can be of some biological significance. All of these observations however merely relate to the presence of the enzyme within the macrophage. Myrvik and Heise (1951) observed that a tuberculostatic substance was present in the serum of immunized rabbits and that this material was similar to lysozyme. Cohn and Wiener (1963a) studied the enzymatic activity of mouse peritoneal macrophages and of normal and activated alveolar macrophages. They found that the lysozyme activity of the alveolar macrophages was very much higher than that of peritoneal macrophages and that the activity of activated alveolar macrophages was considerably higher than that of their normal counterparts. After phagocytosis of heat-killed bacilli there was a marked release of enzymes into the supernatant; this was most striking in the case of lysozyme (Cohn and Wiener, 1963b).

Then in 1967 Heise and Myrvik showed that when rabbit alveolar macrophages were cultivated *in vitro* lysozyme and to a lesser degree acid phosphatase and cathepsin accumulated in the medium. This phenomenon is independent of the serum concentration in the medium and occurs in the absence of phagocytosis.

Evidence on the relationship between lysozyme and macrophages came from another direction in the work of Ossermann and Lawler (1966). These authors studied in detail the physicochemical and immunochemical characteristics of the lysozyme present in the serum and the urine in human patients with monocytic and monomyelocytic leukaemia. They found that the lysozyme present was very similar to normal human lysozyme as found in tears, saliva, serum and leucocytes, but differed quite markedly from egg-white, i.e. avian lysozyme. There was a gross increase in lysozyme in both serum and urine. Since there is in this condition of course a gross increase in monocytes, albeit abnormal monocytes, in marrow and blood, it is reasonable to presume that the lysozyme is produced by the monocytes.

In summary, it is clear that some though not all macrophages contain and probably make significant quantities of lysozyme, that it is of significance in some experimental infections and that it can be released *in vitro* and probably *in vivo*. The intracellular mechanisms of production are obscure. It is not certain whether its release is due to true secretion or simply cellular degeneration and it is very doubtful whether it plays a significant part in the natural response to infection.

Pyrogen

A characteristic of the response of homoiothermic animals to trauma, bacterial or viral infection is fever, the persistent elevation of body temperature. It became clear during the 1950s that the main cause of this during infections is the release of a fever-producing substance or pyrogen by host cells in response to stimulation. Atkins (1960) in reviewing the subject concluded that "granulocytes . . . remain at present the only known source" of pyrogen.

The difficulty about this situation however is that there are several well-known human inflammatory diseases in which fever is marked but the polymorphonuclear response is poor. These are usually granulomatous lesions in which macrophages are prominent in the inflammatory exudate. Tuberculosis is the most obvious.

The first suggestion that cells other than polymorphs produce pyrogen came from Johanovsky (1960) who studied guinea-pigs made hypersensitive to BCG or to Diphtheria-toxoid antitoxin precipitates. When spleen or lymph-node cells from these animals were incubated with the specific toxin a pyrogen was released. Allen (1965a) in rather similar experiments incubated lymph node cells from hypersensitive animals with specific antigen. After incubation for at least 5 h they liberated a pyrogen which produced the brief monophasic febrile response typical of endogenous pyrogen.

The importance of cells other than polymorphs in the febrile response was emphasized by Allen (1965b, c) in a study of fever in agranulocytosis. After rabbits had been rendered hypersensitive to tuberculin they were given a dose of nitrogen mustard to induce agranulocytosis. Animals so treated when challenged with a dose of BCG gave a pyrexial response similar to that of control animals. Similarly their serum contained as much pyrogenic material as serum from control (hypersensitive) animals with normal polymorph counts.

Atkins and Heijn (1965) studied the pyrogenic effect of tuberculin in sensitized rabbits. On incubation of tuberculin with various tissues from rabbits sensitized by an intravenous injection of tuberculin, they could not confirm Johanovsky's finding that lymph node or splenic tissues release a pyrogen but did postulate that cells in the blood were stimulated. A suggested mechanism was that tuberculin makes sensitized monocytes release antibody. This along with antigen acts on polymorphs to make them release pyrogen.

Atkins et al. (1967) showed later that the mechanism was simpler than this. They used rabbits sensitized to tuberculin and obtained alveolar macrophages by washing out their lungs. When these cells were incubated in vitro with tuberculin they released a pyrogen into the supernatant, though they produced it more slowly than polymorphs. Release is almost totally inhibited by puromycin so that it is likely that a true synthetic process is involved. Mononuclear cells from spleen or lymph nodes do not produce a pyrogen under these conditions, but do when activated by staphylococci.

Almost as good evidence was adduced by Bodel and Atkins (1967), that human monocytes release endogenous pyrogen. Patients were studied in whom the proportion of circulating monocytes to polymorphs was very high, as in agranulocytosis and acute monocytic leukaemia; mononuclear cell fractions from normal subjects were also examined. The cells were incubated with staphylococci and material obtained from the supernatant was injected into rabbits, in which it induced pyrexia. After allowing carefully for any possible pyrogen produced by contaminating polymorphs, the authors concluded unequivocally that monocytes were actively producing pyrogen.

Very similar conclusions were arrived at by Hahn et al. (1967) who studied oil-induced peritoneal macrophages. Under a specific set of rather artificial circumstances (incubation for 4 h in exudate fluid and then in potassium free isotonic saline) these cells released a pyrogen. The time curve of the fever produced by this material was similar to the time curve of the fever produced by polymorph pyrogen. However on a quantitative basis macrophages release one fifth as much pyrogen as polymorphs.

It may be concluded that there is now good evidence that macrophages produce and liberate an endogenous pyrogen in vitro in response to specific or non-specific stimuli. The mechanisms of production and release, the chemical nature of the pyrogen and its physiological role in the intact animal are all poorly understood at present.

Interferons

The formation of substances which inhibit viral growth or interferons is a characteristic response of mammalian cells to viral infection. Both peritoneal and alveolar macrophages have been shown to release interferons when grown *in vitro* in presence of various viruses (Glasgow, 1965, 1966; Nagano *et al.*, 1966; Acton and Myrvik, 1966; Subrahmanyan and Mims, 1970). Macrophages from immune mice produce more interferon than those from normal mice and the production is in fact true synthesis since it is inhibited by actinomycin D (Glasgow, 1966). The conditions of inhibition of synthesis of interferons by rabbit peritoneal macrophages suggest that true *de novo* synthesis occurs with sequential transcription and translation of the genetic message (Smith and Wagner, 1966a).

The significance of this *in vitro* work to the situation in the whole animal is at present obscure. Kono and Ho (1965), studied the production of interferon *in vitro* by cells derived from various reticulo-endothelial organs and found that cells from the spleen form interferon more rapidly than those from other organs, and in a manner similar to formation in the intact animal. Some doubt is cast on the significance of macrophage interferons by the demonstration that the interferons formed *in vitro* by rabbit macrophages have molecular weights of 37,000 and 45,000 while those found *in vivo* have molecular weights of 51,000 and 134,000 (Smith and Wagner, 1966b).

In summary there is no doubt that *in vitro* macrophages from several anatomical sites and several species synthesize interferons *in vitro*. The ultrastructural mechanisms involved are not clear and the biological significance doubtful.

Macrophages have been shown to be involved in the formation of some plasma proteins (Phillips and Thorbecke, 1966). These workers produced chimeras by injecting rat marrow into lethally irradiated mice. Donor cells were identified by the presence of marker chromosomes. On culture of RE organs and of peritoneal cells, after 4 weeks in culture βιc globulin and transferrin were found in the culture fluid. The proteins were identified as of rat origin immunologically and the cells in culture identified as of rat origin by marker chromosomes.

The significance of this *in vitro* finding in the whole animal is still obscure and it must be emphasized that the cell cultures were not pure macrophage cultures.

Indirect evidence also exists that cells of the reticuloendothelial system may produce certain clotting factors; reticuloendothelial blockade inhibits production of prothrombin and proconvertin (Slatis, 1958). This is not of course absolute evidence that macrophages actually produce these substances.

Another substance which may be produced by macrophages is amyloid (see Cohen, 1965 for review). This is largely composed of protein with a minor carbohydrate component; in a number of disorders where there is a persistent elevation of serum immunoglobulin levels, amyloid is deposited between the cells of such organs as liver, kidney and spleen, causing cell degeneration by separating cells from their oxygen supply. Amyloid is composed of fine fibrils some 7·5 nm in diameter with a 10 nm periodicity. There is good evidence that at least in liver, amyloid fibrils are found in vacuoles within macrophages (Sorenson et al., 1964). On balance the appearances suggest secretion rather than phagocytosis but this is not certain.

In summary macrophages secrete in vitro enzymes notably lysozyme, pyrogen, interferon and possibly some plasma proteins and amyloid. The production of pyrogen is probably an important biological mechanism; the real significance of the production of the other substances is at present doubtful.

Chapter Nine

THE MACROPHAGE IN IRON
AND LIPID METABOLISM

Macrophages play an important part in the breakdown of red blood cells and the metabolism of their constituents, and in the metabolism of lipids.

It has long been known from morbid anatomical studies in man that in various pathological states red blood cells were sequestered and destroyed in the spleen, and, in conditions of excess red cell breakdown, in the liver.

The site of physiological breakdown of red blood corpuscles was studied by Ehrenstein and Lockner (1958). After the injection into the rabbit of homologous red blood corpuscles labelled with 59Fe 74% of the label was found in the marrow, 2% in the spleen, 8·4% in the liver and 7·9% in the lungs. Similar results were obtained by Miescher (1956) and by Hughes Jones (1961a). Hughes Jones (1961b) and Keene and Jandl (1965) on the other hand studied the rat and found that the marrow played a minor part in the removal of red cells; the marrow played a larger part when it was depleted of blood forming cells, or after carbon blockade of the animal. In a review of previous work Keene and Jandl came to the conclusion that the spleen removed slightly altered and the liver greatly altered cells.

The speed of clearance of red blood cells was explored by Noyes et al. (1960). These authors gave labelled non-viable red cells to humans and rabbits. The average clearance of small amounts was 61% per hour or 20–40 times the normal rate of destruction. The iron from small numbers of red blood cells was utilized rapidly; when large numbers were infused about half of the constituent iron was still retained within the body at two weeks.

The function of the spleen in relation to red blood cells was extensively reviewed by Crosby (1959). The possible ways in which the spleen could act were discussed. Two main mechanisms were postulated. Aged red cells could be removed as a whole by the splenic macrophages, so called "culling" of cells, or iron granules could be removed from red cells without destruction of the red cells, so called "pitting".

The precise mechanism of ingestion of effete red blood corpuscles was poorly understood in the pre-electron microscope era. Possibilities were lysis or fragmentation of the RBC followed by phagocytosis, or phagocytosis of whole cells. Edwards and Simon (1970) have studied the process in some detail in the rat spleen. Phagocytosis was carried out by macrophages in both red and white pulp but not by the endothelial cells lining sinuses. The matrix of the RBC in phagocytic vacuoles becomes heterogeneous and granular; the phagosome membrane then apparently becomes inverted into the red blood cell, so that a series of tunnels of cytoplasm finally invaginates it. Ferritin appears first within the red cell cytoplasm and seems to be able to penetrate the cytoplasmic membrane readily to reach the adjacent cytoplasm. Rhomboidal crystals, probably of haematoidin are sometimes seen. In the rabbit (Simon and Burke, 1970) again whole red cells are ingested. Prominent tunnels of cytoplasm are not formed, probably because the red cell is broken down with less distortion of shape. Myelin figures are however very prominent. In the experimental haemolytic anaemia produced by the administration of phenyl hydrazine the mechanism of red cell breakdown is probably the usual one (Rifkind, 1965).

Lysosomal enzymes have been shown to be involved in the breakdown of RBC (Rifkind, 1966). The relationship of lysosome to phagosome is perhaps best seen in the experimental phagocytosis of RBC by cat alveolar macrophages. Here the macrophage lysosomes have prominent paracrystalline electron dense cores and can be seen fusing with the ingested red blood cells. Discontinuities appear in the membrane of the ingested red blood cell due to the breakdown of its protein components. Thereafter ferritin appears within the phagocytic vesicle (Collet, 1970; Collet and Petrik, 1971a, b).

Early work on the fate of erythrocytes suggested that often red blood cells were destroyed by fragmentation; the fragments were then ingested by the macrophages of spleen and liver (Rous and Robertson, 1917). Essner (1960) demonstrated the engulfment of red cell fragments under rather artificial experimental conditions in the peritoneal cavity. Koyama et al. (1964) and Lawson et al. (1969) observed ingestion of fragments of altered red blood cells in haemolytic anaemia, and Wennberg and Weiss (1968) made similar observations in haemoglobin H disease. On the whole however intravascular fragmentation does not seem to be important in the normal disposal of red blood cells.

The precise relationship of the production of bilirubin to the breakdown of red cells is not quite certain.

It is clear that macrophages break down red blood cells and that bilirubin is partly a product of red blood cell metabolism; it is not however quite clear in what cells bilirubin is formed. With (1968) in a survey of the bile pigments concludes that bilirubin is formed partly in the liver and partly elsewhere, notably in marrow and spleen. The view that macrophages are largely responsible for the formation of bile pigment is strongly supported by the experiments of Dumont et al. (1962) who found that the bilirubin levels in thoracic duct lymph were notably reduced by administration of thorotrast in a dosage sufficient to produce widespread damage to macrophages. While it is possible to interpret the stages of degradation of RBC within macrophages as partly representing the formation of bilirubin, the mode of excretion of bilirubin into the blood stream has not been explored. Moreover it is clear that when haemoglobin is infused in high dosage into the blood of an experimental animal, it can be taken up by hepatic epithelial cells as well as by macrophages; that is while the macrophage is probably the main site for breakdown of aged red blood cells, it is not the only site of disposal of artificially infused haemoglobin (Goldfischer et al., 1970).

Ferritin is certainly produced within macrophages (Richter, 1959; Muir and Golberg, 1961a, b). It appears within lysosomes and also free in the cytoplasm soon after ingestion of red blood cells. Possibly iron is linked on to apoferritin already present within the macrophage. The site of synthesis of the latter substance has not yet been clearly defined. Muir and Golberg (1961a) suggest that it may be either in the cytoplasm or in actual phagocytic vacuoles.

The handling of iron in the bone marrow has been extensively investigated with the electron microscope. A striking feature of marrow is the presence of groups or islets of erythroblasts surrounded by macrophages or reticular cells. The view has been put forward by a group of French workers (see Bessis and Breton-Gorius, 1959, 1962; Koyhani and Bessis, 1969), and Orlic et al. (1965) that ferritin is being passed from macrophage to erythroblast. There is no doubt that their illustrations show ferritin in pinocytotic vesicles at the edge of the erythroblast. Tanaka et al. (1966) on the other hand have pointed out that relatively little ferritin is found on the membrane of the erythroblast and suggest that apoferritin on the surface of the erythroblast picks up iron from the environment.

A different view has been put forward by Berman (1967). Similar islets were identified in the mouse bone marrow. In this case however numerous micropinocytic vesicles were found along the margin of the macrophages, which were heavily loaded with red cell debris, including numbers of paracrystalline inclusions. Berman discussed fully the literature on erythroblastic islets and pointed out that the ferritin might be travelling in either direction.

There is some evidence that as well as acting as stores of iron, macrophages may have a controlling effect on the distribution of iron between haemopoietic and other organs (MacSween and Macdonald, 1969; Macdonald et al., 1969). Macrophages from various sites were shown to take up iron bound to the plasma transport protein transferrin; pulmonary macrophages from anaemic animals took up less iron than normal and macrophages from animals with a turpentine induced pleurisy took up more than normal.

The Macrophage in Lipid Metabolism

The importance of macrophages in lipid metabolism early became evident when Anitschkow (1913) induced atherosclerosis by feeding animals cholesterol and showed that large amounts of lipid accumulated in the liver macrophages.

It has been known for many years that when lipid of various kinds are injected artificially, whether subcutaneously or intravenously they are phagocytosed by the appropriate set of macrophages, like any other particulate material (see Saxl and Donath, 1924; Tompkins, 1946). This is not necessarily relevant to lipid metabolism in the intact animal.

The metabolism of injected lipid by macrophages was studied by Tompkins (1946) who injected cholesterol into the subcutaneous tissues of rats and demonstrated cholesterol esters at the site of injection. After the injection of lipids into the peritoneal cavity, lipid can be demonstrated by histochemical techniques in the draining (diaphragmatic) lymph nodes. After the injection of such substances as cholesterol oleate, sudanophilic material persists in the node longer than after injection of cholesterol. Moreover histochemically a variety of lipids can be demonstrated in the lymph nodes, implying that the original lipid had been metabolically altered, probably in macrophages (French and Morris, 1960; Day and

French, 1961). Subsequently Day and his colleagues showed that macrophages had the ability, under the varying conditions, to hydrolyse and esterify various lipids, both triglycerides and cholesterol. The rate of esterification of cholesterol is reduced by the presence of lecithin (reviewed by Day, 1964). This group of observations on the metabolic properties of macrophages derives significance from the finding that macrophages in arterial walls synthesize phospholipid in experimental atherosclerosis.

The uptake of lipids and lipoproteins *in vitro* was studied electron microscopically by Casley-Smith and Day (1966); corn oil, cholesterol and lipoproteins were presented to the macrophages and their uptake monitored by quantitative radioactive methods. Larger particles of corn oil and cholesterol were taken up in large vesicles, while small lipoprotein particles were taken up in small (100 nm or less) vesicles. The latter process took place as rapidly at 0° as at 37° and was therefore probably not energy dependent. There was no evidence of extracellular degradation of the lipid.

A prominent feature in the atherosclerotic plaque is the presence of numbers of macrophages variously laden with lipid. Leary (1941, 1949) put forward the theory, based purely on light microscopical observation of fixed stained tissues, that macrophages already laden with lipid ("foam cells") migrated from spleen, liver and lungs by the blood stream to the arterial wall and there degenerated, forming the primary cause of the atheromatous plaque. Alternatively the prime occurrence was thrombosis with subsequent digestion and organization of the thrombus; macrophages were involved in the latter process (Duguid, 1946). In an investigation of the pathogenesis of cholesterol atherosclerosis in the rabbit, Rannie and Duguid (1953) demonstrated lipid laden foam cells in the lumen of the blood vessels and showed clumps of such cells attached to the endothelium. They postulated that these cells became incorporated in the wall of the vessel when endothelium grew over them. Duff *et al.* (1957) came to similar conclusions and suggested that the lipid laden monocytes which they saw both on the surface of and deep to the endothelium derived from blood monocytes. Similarly Poole and Florey (1958) demonstrated lipid in endothelial cells and macrophages in such lesions but clearly demonstrated macrophages passing through the endothelium. The phagocytic nature of the macrophages in atheromatous lesions was clearly demonstrated by Duff *et al.* (1954). After intravenous injection of thorotrast this material was found in macrophages in the atheromatous plaques.

The histochemistry of the macrophages in natural and experimental atherosclerosis was studied by Adams and Bayliss (1963) and Adams *et al.*

(1963a). The macrophages contained cholesterol, phospholipid and considerable quantities of oxidative enzymes and phosphatases. The possibility that cholesterol and its esters were fibrogenic was explored by implanting them into rat connective tissue. Cholesterol produces a giant cell granuloma (Adams *et al.*, 1963b); cholesterol, free fatty acids and certain saturated glycerides were notably fibrogenic (Abdulla *et al.*, 1967). The injection of phospholipid makes resolution of the granuloma more rapid (Adams *et al.*, 1963) due to the more rapid resorption of cholesterol (Adams and Morgan, 1967). The implication is that phospholipids may have a protective effect against the progress of atheroma in the arterial wall by stimulating metabolism of cholesterol within macrophages and therefore removal of the cholesterol before it can exert an extensive fibrogenic effect.

The fine structure of experimental atheromatous lesions in the rabbit was studied by Buck (1958) and Parker (1960). The foam cells in these lesions were often so distended with lipid that their nature or indeed origin was obscured. More recently studies have been published of the fine structure of atheromatous lesions in man (Geer *et al.*, 1961), rat (Still and O'Neal, 1962; Hess and Staubli, 1963), dog (Geer, 1965), and rabbit (Parker and Odland, 1966a, b).

There are considerable interspecies differences. But while some foam cells clearly derive from smooth muscle (Geer, 1965; Parker and Odland, 1966a, b) monocytes or macrophages can clearly be seen sticking to endothelium (Still and O'Neal, 1962; Hess and Staubli, 1963) and accumulating lipid, digesting and releasing the lipid into the circulation. Similar foam cells like lipid-laden macrophages are seen in irradiated arteries (Kirkpatrick, 1967). Here also some foam cells may be derived from smooth muscle cells. An excellent recent study of the origin of foam cells in atherosclerosis is that of Cookson (1971). In rabbits with moderate hypercholesterolaemia foam cells of two types were found. One type characteristically contained numerous cytoplasmic fibrils and was surrounded by a basement membrane; this was probably a smooth muscle cell. The other, a macrophage, had numerous cytoplasmic processes, contained many cytoplasmic inclusions, gave a positive acid phosphatase reaction and was metalophilic.

In a number of uncommon human diseases there is abnormal storage of lipids or polysaccharides in macrophages, usually in large secondary lysosomes, in most cases due to congenital deficiency of an enzyme necessary for the metabolism of the substance concerned. The most common of these is probably Gaucher's disease where a glycolipid cerebroside is stored as tubular structures 25–70 nm in diameter. Wide variations in the ultrastructure of the inclusions occur in different lesions, probably related at least in part to variations in processing in different laboratories (see Brunning, 1970; Resibois *et al.*, 1970 for reviews). Artificial storage disorders can be produced in experimental animals by the repeated injection of substances which macrophages cannot metabolize, for instance methylcellulose (Teoh, 1961).

Xanthomas are skin lesions composed largely of lipid containing macrophages. These lesions occur in human subjects, usually in the presence of elevated plasma lipid levels, and in rabbits fed high fat diets. In each case the component cells are usually macrophages, but are occasionally recognizable vascular pericytes. They contain vacuoles, myelin figures and cholesterol clefts; lipoprotein aggregates are sometimes visible in the blood vessel walls (Imaeda, 1960; Parker and Odland, 1969; Zemel *et al.*, 1969).

It has long been known that there is some relationship between steroid (particularly oestrogen) secretion and macrophage activity. Nicol (1932, 1935) showed in experimental animals that the number of macrophages in the endometrium fell after ovariectomy and increased again after oestrogen injection. The number of macrophages was maximal at proestrus (when endogenous oestrogen secretion was high) and at metestrus (at the time of endometrial breakdown). Whole body reticulo-endothelial function as measured by the uptake of congo red after intravenous injection is increased in human pregnancy; similar increase in uptake of colloids from the circulation of experimental animals occur at proestrus and during pregnancy (when oestrogen levels are high) and at metoestrus, when there is marked degeneration of the endometrium (see Vernon-Roberts, 1969 for an excellent review of this field). It is clear that high doses of oestrogens do increase the rate of clearance of colloids from the blood stream; this is partly due to proliferation of Kupffer cells (Kelly *et al.*, 1962). However the techniques used to measure colloid clearance measure other things than macrophage function and it is far from certain at present whether oestrogens have a direct effect on macrophages.

There is some evidence that reticuloendothelial cells presumably macrophages can play a part in steroid metabolism. Berliner *et al.* (1964) showed that adrenal R.E. cells can add a hydroxyl group to cortisol in position 17 of the steroid ring and the same group (Nabors *et al.*, 1967) have more recently shown that hepatic R.E. cells can reduce ring A of corticosteroids thus lowering the level of anti-inflammatory steroid activity. The chemically reduced steroids which result can induce fever, lower blood cholesterol, and have anaesthetic properties.

Chapter Ten

THE CYTOLOGY OF NEOPLASMS OF MACROPHAGE LINEAGE

As stated in Chapter Three, experimental studies provide strong evidence for the view that in laboratory rodents, macrophages in most sites derive largely from circulating monocytes of recent bone marrow origin. In human lymphoreticular tissues the position is a little less straightforward. Many pathologists using light microscopy describe the existence of a large cell some 20 μm in diameter; when stained by conventional light microscopic techniques its cytoplasm is pale, and its nucleus large and pale, with a coarse open network of chromatin. This cell type has been described as a "reticulum" cell or reticular cell. The latter term is quite ambiguous and should not be applied to such cells.

Some critical observers (e.g. Gall, 1958) have denied the existence of such a cell. Ultrastructural observations of human lymphoreticular tissue (Bernhard and Leplus, 1964; Mori and Lennert, 1969) show however that there are some cells in such tissue which cannot be clearly categorized as lymphocytes, macrophages or fibroblasts. These range from 15–30 μm in diameter and are often though not always longer in one axis than another. The nucleus has an open meshwork of chromatin and sometimes a nucleolus. The cytoplasmic sap is dense in the smaller cells and pale in the larger cells and contains considerable numbers of ribosomes, many of which are aggregated into polysomes. Mitochondria are usually few and rather small and there are few or no lysosomes. Membrane systems, both rough and smooth granular endoplasmic reticulum are rather poorly developed. The cell surface, particularly that of the larger cells, may show a moderate number of cytoplasmic processes. It is convenient to call such cells reticulum cells, and to express their wide range of size by describing them as small and large reticulum cells. Intermediate forms are found between such cells and macrophages but there is no conclusive evidence that such a transformation commonly occurs. Moreover neoplastic cells of this type often have the ability to lay down true collagen. The term "reticulum cell" then refers to a heterogeneous group of cells, many of which may be macrophage precursors and some of which may be able to produce collagen. There is no good evidence that under normal conditions they can divide frequently (Fig. 47).

Neoplasms of Macrophage Lineage

It is uncommon in the extreme to find neoplasms composed of mature differentiated macrophages. On the other hand a number of fairly common human neoplastic conditions are said to arise as neoplasms of the "reticulum cell".

Experimental neoplasms have been induced in the reticuloendothelial system of animals by the repeated injection of foreign substances. Gillman et al. (1949) produced a hyperplasia of reticuloendothelial elements in the liver by the repeated injection of trypan blue. Two types of neoplasms subsequently developed—a reticulum cell sarcoma which was only locally invasive and a spindle cell sarcoma which invaded widely and metastasized.

The injection of radioactive thorium dioxide ("Thorotrast") as a radiological contrast medium provided an inadvertent pathological model in the human subject (reviewed by Silva da Horta, 1967; Grampa, 1971). At the sites of deposition of the material there was a granulomatous reaction, followed after many years by neoplastic change. Among the commonest neoplasms were reticulum cell sarcomas and sarcomas of the cells lining liver sinusoids, though whether of the macrophages or the endothelial cells is not clear.

Two neoplasms occur commonly in the human subject which may reasonably be regarded as neoplasms of reticulum cells—Hodgkin's disease and reticulum cell sarcoma. (See Rappaport, 1966 for an authoritative review.) Both affect principally the lymph nodes, spleen and liver but may spread to other tissues; both are malignant. Their ultrastructure has been illustrated by Bernhard and Leplus (1964) and Mori and Lennert (1969). In Hodgkin's disease the prominent and probably the neoplastic cell resembles a large reticulum cell as defined above, varying in size from 10–40 μm. The smaller cells have a single nucleus, the larger cells have two nuclei often paired, with prominent nucleoli. The cytoplasm has a prominent component of free ribosomes but fairly scanty granular endoplasmic reticulum. The mitochondria are small and there are usually one or two small membrane bound dense bodies, probably lysosomes. There are sometimes but not always prominent microvilli at the cell surface (Figs 48, 49 and 50) but characteristically these cells are accompanied by varying numbers of eosinophils and lymphocytes and by the laying down of fibrous tissue. In reticulum cell sarcoma the component neoplastic cells are similar to the above. Any individual neoplasm is commonly composed of either small or large reticulum cells. Often individual cells are surrounded by a basket work of very fine collagen. Reticulum cell sarcomas occur much more often than would be expected in human subjects taking immunosuppressive drugs to allow the survival of grafts.

Much less commonly neoplasms of differentiated macrophages occur. Fibrous nodules occur in the skin composed largely of histiocytes; most of these are not truly neoplastic. Similar nodules of rather yellowish colour in which the histiocytes contain large amounts of lipid are known as xanthomas; these are usually but not always accompanied by elevated lipid levels (see Chapter Eight). Again these are probably not truly neoplastic. Other rare neoplasms arise as nodules in the skin and are composed of cells which look rather like epithelioid macrophages. With the electron microscope these cells are seen to have numerous pseudopodia often interdigitating; the cytoplasm contains prominent endoplasmic reticulum and dense bodies, probably lysosomes. Such lesions recur and may metastasize and kill the patient. The term applied to these by Enzinger (1970) and Mackenzie (1971) is epithelioid sarcoma. It seems likely that they are true malignant neoplasms of differentiated macrophages. A lesion entitled "fibroxanthosarcoma" by Merkow, Frich *et al.* (1971) appears to be similar in nature; here however many of the neoplastic histiocytes contained considerable amounts of lipid and there were neoplastic fibroblasts in the lesion.

In addition to these localized neoplasms, a number of uncommon related human diseases occur in which the tissues are diffusely infiltrated by histiocytes; the overall term for this group of conditions is histiocytosis. The lesions are probably neoplastic and range in clinical behaviour from the rapidly lethal to the relatively benign. The ultrastructure of these lesions has been reported by various authors (Basset *et al.*, 1965; Cancella *et al.*, 1967; de Man, 1968; Morales *et al.*, 1969; Shamoto, 1970). The component macrophages vary in degree of differentiation but contain curious cytoplasmic inclusions, elongated and probably tubular with an electron dense core. Their nature is not certain but they resemble the inclusions seen in the

Langerhans cells of skin and those seen in micropinocytosis vermiformis. These conditions can probably be regarded as diffuse neoplastic proliferations of macrophage-like cells.

It must be emphasized that the derivation of all of these conditions requires much further ultrastructural study.

Chapter Eleven

MACROPHAGE-LIKE CELLS

It has been the theme of this book that macrophages are a closely related family of cells largely derived from bone marrow mononuclear cells, normally highly phagocytic and similar in their cytochemical and ultra-structural pattern and either actually or potentially freely moving from a common pool. There are a number of cell types in various environments in the body which resemble macrophages in many ways but which while they can be stimulated to phagocytosis are not always freely phagocytic and which do not form part of the common macrophage pool in the body. The ultrastructure of these will be considered briefly in this chapter in particular relation to their phagocytic function. They are: The great alveolar cell of the lung. The mesothelial cell. The Sertoli cell. The epithelial reticular cell of the thymus. The osteoclast and the chondroclast. They can be regarded as sequestrated phagocytes, phagocytic in varying degree but only in relation to their own secluded environment.

The Great Alveolar Epithelial Cell

The long standing controversy on the origin of the phagocytic cells of the pulmonary alveolus has been considered elsewhere. It is now generally accepted that most of these cells under most circumstances are true macrophages, derived ultimately in the main from the marrow but partly from the interstitial tissues of the lung. However there must always be a few shed epithelial cells in the alveolar cavity and this proportion may increase under some abnormal circumstances. The purpose of the present section is to consider the structure and function of the great alveolar cells, or granular pneumonocytes.

The structure of the great alveolar epithelial cell has been well reviewed by Sorokin (1966, see this author for fuller bibliography). It is a large cell sometimes packed into a niche in the wall of the alveolus, sometimes bulging into the lumen of the alveolus. It is distinguished from the squamous alveolar cells by its size, large osmiophilic inclusions, prominent mitochondria and small microvilli on its free surface (Fig. 51) (Low, 1952; Karrer, 1958; Schulz, 1959). The prominent osmiophilic inclusions range in size from 0·1–1 μ in diameter, are delineated by membrane and have a myelin-like structure; they contain sudanophilic lipid and glyco-protein and are probably discharged into the alveoli as the surfactant which keeps the alveolar surface tension down (Klaus et al., 1962; Bensch et al., 1964; Hatasa and Nakamura, 1965) (Fig. 45). Considerable amounts of acid phosphatase are present at the edge of the cytoplasmic inclusions (Corrin et al., 1969). There is good EM autoradiographic evidence that after injection of tritiated palmitate it is incorporated by great alveolar cells in their osmiophilic inclusions, clear evidence of active secretion (Askin and Kuhn, 1971).

Great alveolar cells are only poorly phagocytic when fixed on the alveolar wall (Low and Sampaio, 1957). It seems possible however that when shed into the alveolus they may be more active. Studies are fre-quently carried out on populations of cells washed out from the lung; such preparations must inevitably contain varying numbers of great alveolar cells, distinguishable only by electron microscopy.

The Mesothelial Cell

In many of the older accounts of the free macrophages of serosal cavities it is suggested that mesothelial cells are a possible precursor of macro-phages (see Cappell, 1929). Mesothelial cells are flattened cells, usually joined to their neighbours by desmosomes and with numerous fairly straight finger-like processes 0·5–1 μm long on their serosal surfaces. The cytoplasm has rather scanty rough endoplasmic reticulum and other membrane systems as compared to the macrophage; along the serosal surface of the cell are numerous micropinocytic vesicles some 50–100 nm in diameter (Fig. 52). There are no larger vacuoles such as are found in the macrophage, and the prominent ectoplasmic zone of cytoplasm which is characteristic of the macrophage is absent (Carr, 1967). Felix and Dalton (1956) studied the ability of mesothelial cells to ingest particles and pointed out that they could not ingest such large structures as melanin granules, but are able to ingest such small particles as thorotrast, that is they are capable of micropinocytosis but not of true phagocytosis.

It seems likely however that under certain abnormal circumstances mesothelial cells can become actively phagocytic, for instance after stimulation of the pleural cavity with the irritant fat soluble dye Sudan III (Young, 1928). The converse may occur. When a millipore chamber is implanted into the peritoneal cavity, the free peritoneal cells settle on it and within a few days become serosal cells (Eskeland, 1967).

The Sertoli Cell

The cells of Sertoli lie between the germ cells of the testis; their main function is to provide a milieu for intracellular maturation of spermatids. They are pyramidal in shape with the apex pointing into the lumen of the tubule; the nucleus characteristically shows an indentation. The long axis of the nucleus may be parallel to or perpendicular to the basement membrane of the tubule. Acid phosphatase and other lysosomal enzymes are demonstrable in the cytoplasm (Niemi *et al.*, 1962; Niemi and Kormano, 1965).

As seen with the electron microscope (Bawa, 1963; Carr *et al.*, 1968) normal Sertoli cells have a mass of cytoplasm at the periphery of the seminiferous tubule with a process extending down to the lumen of the tubule. The cytoplasmic matrix tends to be notably more dense than that of surrounding germ cells. Both granular and agranular endoplasmic reticulum are present in moderate amounts; each cell profile usually shows several lysosomal dense bodies, commonly homogeneous in structure and rather similar to macrophage lysosomes (Fig. 53). Flaps of cytoplasm are present on the luminal border of the cell; these enclose shallow invaginations of the cell surface. Spermatid heads are found in clusters embedded in the cytoplasm of the Sertoli cell as part of normal sperm maturation. The mechanics at an organelle or biochemical level of what goes on within the Sertoli cell are quite unknown but it seems very likely that small fragments of spermatid material are ingested by the Sertoli cell. Under various abnormal circumstances the Sertoli cell can actually phagocytose germ cells.

The phagocytic properties of the Sertoli cell were strikingly demonstrated by Clegg and Macmillan (1965) who injected carbon suspensions into the tubules and found that they were taken up by the Sertoli cell. After similar injections of a colloidal iron suspension particles were seen to be taken up into phagocytic vacuoles in the Sertoli cells (Carr *et al.*, 1968).

The Epithelial Reticular Cell of the Thymus

The presence of distinctive cells of epithelial origin in the thymus was strongly suggested by the observation by Metcalf and Ishidate (1961) of a separate group of cells staining positively by the periodic acid Schiff technique and therefore containing glycoprotein. They were characterized as a distinctive group by electron microscopy (Palumbi and Millonig, 1961; Weiss, 1963b; Clark, 1963). The earlier literature on these cells is reviewed by Toro (1967) and the ultrastructure by Carr (1970).

The epithelial reticular cells are large cells which fall not very precisely into two groups, cortical and medullary with considerable overlap between them. In both sites they form the essential framework of the organ and their processes abut on one another being related by desmosomes.

The cortical cells give off numerous processes which form a functionally incomplete sheath round the blood vessels. The cytoplasm of these cells contains some ergastoplasm and a few small secretory granules. The prominent feature of the cytoplasm, however, is the presence of numerous tonofibrils similar in structure to the keratinous fibrils of squamous epithelial cells (Fig. 54).

The medullary cells on the other hand have a much more obvious endoplasmic reticulum and Golgi apparatus and contain numerous membrane bound granules. Their most characteristic feature is the presence of intracellular vacuoles 1 μm or more in diameter from whose walls arise microvilli and even cilia. These cells hypertrophy after involution of the thymus (Ito and Hoshino, 1962; Gad and Clark, 1968). They also incorporated administered radioactive sulphate (Clark, 1968). Clark puts forward evidence that during acute involution of the thymus "lymphopoiesis and sulphate incorporation . . . correlated linearly over a wide range in variation, providing circumstantial evidence to support the hypothesis that medullary epithelial cells secrete a sulfated mucoid lymphopoietic hormone".

Medullary epithelial cells also play a large part in the formation of the curious degenerate cellular whorls known as Hassall's corpuscles. In addition it has been suggested (Toro, 1967; Cowan and Sorenson, 1964; Blackburn and Miller, 1964a, b) that epithelial reticular cells are phagocytic at least toward lymphocytes. No unequivocal evidence of phagocytosis was noted by Gad and Clark (1968).

The thymic epithelial reticular cell therefore is a cell which may be confused with a macrophage and probably has some phagocytic activity within the thymus. It probably has at least one more important function, the secretion of a lymphopoietic hormone.

The Osteoclast

The presence of large multinucleate cells along the edges of bone trabeculae was first noticed by Kolliker (1872). The older work has been well reviewed by Hancox (1956). The cells are 20–100 μm in diameter and may contain up to 100 nuclei. The cytoplasm is often in part basophilic but may contain glycoprotein inclusions. A wide spectrum of lysosomal enzymes occurs in the cytoplasm very similar to those found in the macrophage at other sites and including acid phosphatase, β-galactosidase, β-glucuronidase, phosphoamidase and aminopeptidase. The acid phosphatase is often present in a distinct junctional zone next to bone (Burstone, 1959; Tonna, 1961, review by Vaes, 1969).

The fine structure of the osteoclast has been studied by Scott and Pease (1956), Cameron and Robinson (1958), Hancox and Boothroyd (1961), Gonzales and Karnovsky (1961) and Anderson and Parker (1966). Their accounts are in general agreement.

The cells have a markedly ruffled border apposed to the bone surface. Between the processes of cytoplasm lie numerous invaginations in which lie crystals of bone salt (Figs 55 and 56). These may also be seen in vacuoles within the cell. In sites of cartilage resorption at the epiphyses quite large pieces of chondrified material may be seen. It is presumed that some secretion of material, probably lysosomal, occurs but no convincing ultrastructural evidence of it has yet been produced. In cartilage resorption ordinary macrophages also are involved (Anderson and Parker, 1967).

When grown *in vitro* the cytoplasmic membrane of osteoclasts next to resorbing bone shows numerous small bristles 15–20 nm long; the cytoplasmic membrane at these sites probably indents to form coated vesicles. The development of the ruffled border is markedly inhibited by the presence of the thyroid hormone calcitonin in the medium; this suggests that this hormone inhibits bone resorption by a direct action on osteoclasts (Kallio *et al.*, 1971, 1972).

Scott (1967) has brought forward valuable evidence of the similarity of the osteoclast to macrophages at other sites, showing that they contain membrane bound dense bodies similar to those of other macrophages. Some of these are small and homogeneous with a finely granular substructure, like the primary lysosomes of macrophages elsewhere. Others are larger and more pleomorphic and are clearly residual bodies. Doty *et al.* (1968) have shown that these bodies contain acid phosphatase.

There can now be little doubt that osteoclasts do phagocytose bone. *In vitro* they move like macrophages with a ruffled edge and numerous vesicles (Hancox and Boothroyd, 1961). These authors caution however that it is not yet quite certain whether they cause the resorption of bone as opposed to scavenging bone that has already and for other reasons been resorbed.

The origin of the osteoclast has been the origin of much controversy; possible progenitors including the monocyte, the lymphocyte, the osteocyte and the chondrocyte. Tonna (1961, 1963) has studied the labelling pattern in young animals and after fractures, after the injection of tritiated thymidine. Mature osteoclasts do not label readily; the precursors were probably mononuclear cells, interpreted by this author as osteoblasts of varying maturity. Fischman and Hay (1962) studied regeneration of the amputated leg of a newt by autoradiography after the administration of tritiated thymidine; four to five days after the amputation there was a rapid influx of labelled polymorphs and monocytes. At the 8th day 90% of the osteoclasts were labelled. Generally not all of the nuclei in a given osteoclast were labelled. Quite soon thereafter no more labelled cells were seen, suggesting that the life span of these osteoclasts was not much more than ten days. Again mitosis was not seen in osteoclasts. Jee and Nolan (1963) injected bone charcoal into the nutrient artery of the rabbit femur and examined the pattern of phagocytosis of the carbon in sections of the bone. Carbon was seen initially in blood vessels, then in macrophages and only much later in osteoclasts. The reasonable conclusion from the above work is that osteoclasts derive probably by cell fusion from mononuclear phagocytic cells, of ultimate bone marrow origin; these cells are probably in fact macrophages, though whether they are quite identical to macrophages elsewhere is not certain. The immature precursor cell of the osteoclast in situations of rapid bone turnover may bear a considerable resemblance to that of the osteoblast.

It is not certain whether a distinct cell type, the chondroclast is responsible for the breakdown of cartilage. The findings of Anderson and Parker (1967) suggest that macrophages and osteoclasts are responsible for the breakdown of cartilage and do not support the notion that there is a separate chondroclast.

REFERENCES

Abdulla, Y. H., Adams, C. W. M. and Morgan, R. S. (1967). *J. Path. Bact.* **94,** 63–71.

Acton, J. D. and Myrvik, Q. N. (1966). *J. Bact.* **91,** 2300–2304.

Adam, W. S. (1966). *Nature, Lond.* **211,** 771–772.

Adams, C. W. M. and Bayliss, O. B. (1963). *J. Path. Bact.* **85,** 113–119.

Adams, C. W. M. and Morgan, R. S. (1967). *J. Path. Bact.* **94,** 73–76.

Adams, C. W. M., Bayliss, O. B. and Ibrahim, M. Z. M. (1963). *J. Path. Bact.* **86,** 421–430.

Adams, C. W. M., Bayliss, O. B., Ibrahim, M. Z. M. and Webster, M. W. (1963). *J. Path. Bact.* **86,** 431–436.

Adlersberg, L., Singer, J. M. and Ende, E. (1969). *J. reticuloendothel. Soc.* **6,** 536–560.

Adrian, E. K. and Walker, B. W. (1962). *J. Neuropath. exp. Neurol.* **21,** 597–609.

Albrecht, R. M., Hinsdill, R. D., Sandok, P. L., Mackenzie, A. B. and Sachs, L. B. (1972). *Expl. Cell Res.* **70,** 230–232.

Alexander, P. (1968). *Prog. exp. Tumor Res.* **10,** 22–71.

Allen, I. V. (1965a). *J. Path. Bact.* **89,** 481–494.

Allen, I. V. (1965b). *J. Path. Bact.* **89,** 495–502.

Allen, I. V. (1965c). *Immunology* **8,** 396–405.

Allen, J. M., Brieger, E. M. and Rees, R. J. W. (1965). *J. Path. Bact.* **89,** 301–306.

Allen, J. M., and Cook, G. M. W. (1970). *Expl. Cell Res.* **59,** 105–116.

Allison, A. C., Harrington, J. S. and Birbeck, N. (1966). *J. exp. Med.* **124,** 141–153.

Allison, A. C. (1970). *In* "The Mononuclear Phagocyte" (van Furth, R., ed.), Blackwell, London.

Amos, H. E. and Lachmann, P. J. (1970). *Immunology* **18,** 269–278.

Anderson, C. E. and Parker, J. (1967). *J. Bone Joint Surg.* **48A,** 899–914.

Anitschkow, N. (1913). *Münch. med. Wchnschr.* **2,** 2255–2258.

Anton, E. and Brandes, D. (1969). *J. Ultrastruct. Res.* **26,** 69–84.

Aoki, T., Hammerling, U., de Harven, E., Boyse, E. A. and Old, L. J. (1969). *J. exp. Med.* **130,** 979–1001.

Argyris, B. A. (1968). *J. exp. Med.* **128,** 459–467.

Armstrong, J. A. and Hart, P. D'A. (1971). *J. exp. Med.* **134,** 713–740.

Aronow, R., Danon, D., Shahar, A. and Aronson, M. (1964) *J. exp. Med.* **120,** 943–954.

Aronson, M. (1963). *J. exp. Med.* **118,** 1083–1088.

Aronson, M. and Elberg, S. (1962). *Proc. nat. Acad. Sci., U.S.A.* **48,** 208–214.

Aronson, M. and Shahar, M. (1965). *Exp. Cell Res.* **38,** 133–143.

Aschoff, L. (1924). *In* "Lectures in Pathology", pp. 1–33. Hoeber, New York.

Ashworth, G. T., Diluzio, N. R. and Riggi, S. J. (1963). *Expl. mol. Path.* *Suppl.* **1**, 83–103.

Askin, F. B. and Kuhn, C. (1971). *Lab. Invest.* **25**, 260–268.

Askonas, B. A. and Rhodes, J. M. (1965). *Nature, Lond.* **205**, 470–474.

Askonas, B. A., Auzins, I. and Unanue, E. R. (1968). *Bull. Soc. Chim. Biol.* **50**, 1113–1128.

Aterman, K. (1963). "The Liver", Vol. 1, pp. 61–136. (Rouiller, Ch., ed.) Academic Press, New York and London.

Atkins, E. (1960). *Physiol. Rev.* **40**, 580–646.

Atkins, E. and Heijn, C. (1965). *J. exp. Med.* **122**, 207–235.

Atkins, E., Bodel, P. and Francis, L. (1967). *J. exp. Med.* **126**, 357–384.

Axline, S. and Cohn, Z. A. (1970). *J. exp. Med.* **131**, 1239–1260.

Bailiff, R. N. (1963). *Ann. N.Y. Acad. Sci.* **88**, 3–13.

Baldridge, C. W. and Gerard, R. W. (1933). *Am. J. Physiol.* **103**, 235–236.

Ballantyne, B. (1967). *In* "The Reticuloendothelial System and Atherosclerosis" (Diluzio, N. R. & Paoletti, R., eds), pp. 121–132. Plenum Press, New York.

Ballantyne, B. (1968). *J. reticuloendothel. Soc.* **5**, 399–411.

Ballantyne, B. and Burwell, R. G. (1965). *Nature, Lond.* **206**, 1122–1125.

Balner, H. (1963). *Transplantation* **1**, 217–233.

Barka, T., Schaffner, F., and Popper, H. (1961). *Lab. Invest.* **10**, 589–607.

Barnes, J. M. (1941). *Br. J. exp. Path.* **21**, 264–275.

Bartfeld, H., and Kelley, R. (1968). *J. Immunol.* **100**, 1000–1005.

Basset, F., Nezelof, C., Mallet, R. and Turiaf, J. (1965). *C. r. hebd. Séanc. Acad. Sci. Paris.* **26**, 5719–5720.

Bawa, S. R. (1963). *J. Ultrastr. Res.* **9**, 459–474.

Beard, J. W., and Rous, P. (1934). *J. exp. Med.* **59**, 593–607.

Bennett, B. (1966). *Am. J. Path.* **48**, 165–181.

Bennett, B. and Bloom, B. R. (1967). *Transplantation* **5**, 996–1000.

Bennet, B., Old, L. J. and Boyse, E. A. (1964). *Transplantation* **2**, 183–202.

Bennett, H. S., Luft, J. H. and Hampton, J. C. (1959). *Am. J. Physiol.* **196**, 381–390.

Bennett, W. E. and Cohn, Z. A. (1966). *J. exp. Med.* **123**, 145–160.

Bensch, K., Schaefer, K. and Avery, M. E. (1964). *Science, N.Y.* **145**, 1318–1319.

Berken, A. and Benacerraf, B. (1966). *J. exp. Med.* **123**, 119–144.

Berliner, D. L., Nabors, C. J. and Dougherty, T. F. (1964). *J. reticuloendothel. Soc.* **1**, 1–17.

Berman, L. (1966). *Lab. Invest.* **15**, 1084–1099.

Berman, I. (1967). *J. Ultrastruct. Res.* **17**, 291–313.

Bernhard, W. and Leplus, R. (1964). "Fine Structure of the Normal and Malignant Human Lymph Node". Macmillan (Pergamon), New York.

Berry, L. J. and Spies, T. D. (1949). *Medicine* **28**, 239–300.

Bertalanffy, F. D. (1964a), *Int. Rev. Cytol.* **16**, 234–328.

Bertalanffy, F. D. (1964b), *Int. Rev. Cytol.* **17**, 214–297.

Bessis, M. and Breton-Gorius, J. (1959). *J. biophys. biochem. Cytol.* **6**, 231–236.

Bessis, M. and Breton-Gorius, J. (1962). *Blood* **19**, 635–653.

Bessis, M. and Thiery, J. P. (1961). *Int. Rev. Cytol.* **12,** 199–241.

Biozzi, G., Benacerraf, B. and Halpern, B. N. (1953). *Br. J. exp. Path.* **34,** 441–457.

Birbeck, M. S. C. and Carter, R. L. (1972). *Int. J. Cancer* **9,** 249–257.

Bishop, D. C., Pisciotta, A. V. and Abramoff, P. (1967). *J. Immunol.* **99,** 751–759.

Black, M. M., Opler, S. R. and Speer, F. D. (1955). *Surg. Gynaec. Obstet.* **100,** 543–551.

Black, M. M., Opler, S. R. and Speer, F. D. (1956). *Surg. Gynaec. Obstet.* **102,** 599–603.

Blackburn, W. R. and Miller, J. F. A. P. (1967a). *Lab. Invest.* **16,** 66–83.

Blackburn, W. R. and Miller, J. F. A. P. (1967b). *Lab. Invest.* **16,** 833–846.

Blanden, R. V. (1968). *J. reticuloendothel. Soc.* **5,** 179–202.

Blinzinger, K. and Kreutzberg, G. (1968). *Z. Zellforsch. Mikrosk. Anat.* **85,** 145–157.

Bloom, W. (1938). *In* "Handbook of Hematology" (Downey, H., ed.), pp. 373–437. Hoeber, New York.

Boak, J. K., Christie, G. H., Ford, W. C. and Howard, J. G. (1968). *Proc. roy. Soc. B.* **169,** 307–327.

Bodel, P. and Atkins, E. (1967). *New Engl. J. Med.* **276,** 1002–1008.

Bonicke, R., Fasske, E. and Themann, H. (1963). *Klin. Wochschr.* **41,** 753–768.

Botham, S. K. and Holt, P. F. (1968). *J. Path. Bact.* **96,** 443–453.

Boughton, B. and Spector, W. G. (1963). *J. Path. Bact.* **85,** 371–381.

Bowden, D. H., Davies, E. and Wyatt, J. P. (1968). *Arch. Path.* **86,** 667–670.

Boyden, S. V. (1962). *J. exp. Med.* **115,** 453–466.

Boyden, S. V. (1964). *Int. Rev. exp. Path.* **2,** 311–356.

Boyden, S. V. and Sorkin, E. (1961). *Immunology* **4,** 244–252.

Braunstein, H. and Schmalzl, F. (1970). *In* "The Mononuclear Phagocyte", pp. 62–81 (van Furth, R. ed.). Blackwell, London.

Braunstein, H., Freiman, D. G. and Gall, E. A. (1958). *Cancer* **11,** 829–837.

Breathnach, A. S. (1964). *J. Anat. Lond.* **98,** 265–270.

Breathnach, A. S. (1965). *Int. Rev. Cytol.* **18,** 1–37.

Briggs, R. S., Perillie, P. E. and Finch, S. C. (1966). *J. Histochem. Cytochem.* **14,** 167–170.

Brooks, R. E. and Siegel, B. Z. (1966). *Blood* **27,** 687–705.

Brucher, H. (1958). *In* "Physiology and Pathology of Leucocytes" (Braunsteiner, F. & Zucker Franklin, D., eds). Grune and Stratton, New York.

Brumfitt, W. and Glynn, A. A. (1961). *Br. J. exp. Path.* **42,** 408–423.

Brunning, R. D. (1970). *Human Pathology* **1,** 99–124.

Bruyn de P. P. H. (1945). *Anat. Rec.* **93,** 295–315.

Buck, R. C. (1958). *Am. J. Path.* **34,** 897–909.

Burke, J. S. and Simon, G. T. (1970a). *Am. J. Path.* **58,** 127–155.

Burke, J. S. and Simon, G. T. (1970b). *Am. J. Path.* **58,** 157–181.

Burkel, W. E. and Low, F. N. (1965). *Am. J. Anat.* **118,** 769–784.

Burstone, M. S. (1959). *Ann. N.Y. Acad. Sci.* **85,** 431–444.

Buyukozer, I., Mutlu, K. S. and Pepe, F. A. (1965). *Am. J. Anat.* **117,** 385–416.

Cameron, D. A. and Robinson, R. A. (1958). *J. Bone Jt. Surg.* **40A,** 414–418.

Cancella, P. A., Lahey, E. and Carnes, W. H. (1967). *Cancer* **20,** 1986–1991.

Cappell, D. F. (1929). *J. Path. Bact.* **33,** 429–452.

Carr, I. (1962). *J. Path. Bact.* **83,** 443–448.

Carr, I. (1967a). *Z. Zellforsch. Mikrosk. Anat.* **80,** 534–555.

Carr, I. (1967b). *J. Path. Bact.* **94,** 323–330.

Carr, I. (1968a). *Z. Zellforsch. Mikrosk. Anat.* **89,** 328–354.

Carr, I. (1968b). *Z. Zellforsch. Mikrosk. Anat.* **89,** 355–370.

Carr, I. (1970). *Int. Rev. Cytol.* **27,** 283–348.

Carr, I. (1972). *J. Anat. Lond.* **112,** 383–389.

Carr, I., Clarke, J. A. and Salsbury, A. J. (1969). *J. Microsc.* **89,** 105–111.

Carr, I., Clegg, E. J. and Meek, G. A. (1968). *J. Anat. Lond.,* **102,** 501–509.

Carr, I., Everson, G., Rankin, A. and Rutherford, J. (1970). *Z. Zellforsch Mikrosk. Anat.* **105,** 339–349.

Carr, I. and Williams, M. A. (1967). *In* "The Reticulo-endothelial System and Atherosclerosis" (Diluzio, N. R. and Paoletti, R. eds). pp. 98–107. Plenum Press, New York.

Carr, K. and Carr, I. (1970). *Z. Zellforsch. Mikrosck. Anat.* **105,** 234–241.

Carrel, A. and Ebeling, A. H. (1922). *J. exp. Med.* **36,** 365–377.

Carrel, A. and Ebeling, A. H. (1926). *J. exp. Med.* **44,** 285–305.

Carson, M. E. and Dannenberg, A. M. (1965). *J. Immunol.* **94,** 99–104.

Carstein, P. M. (1961). *Z. Zellforsch Mikrosk. Anat.* **54,** 252–261.

Carter, R. L. and Gershon, R. K. (1966). *Am. J. Path.* **49,** 637–655.

Carter, R. L. and Gershon, R. K. (1967). *Am. J. Path.* **50,** 203–217.

Casley-Smith, J. R. (1964). *Q. Jl exp. Physiol.* **49,** 365–383.

Casley-Smith, J. R. (1965). *Br. J. exp. Path.* **46,** 35–49.

Casley-Smith, J. R. (1969). *J. Miscroscopy* **90,** 15–30.

Casley-Smith, J. R. and Day, A. J. (1966). *Q. Jl exp. Physiol.* **51,** 1–10.

Casley-Smith, J. R. and Reade, P. C. (1965). *Br. J. exp. Path.* **46,** 473–480.

Catanzaro, P. J., Graham, R. C., Jr. and Schwartz, H. J. (1969). *J. Immunol.* **103,** 618–621.

Cayeux, P., Panijel, P., Cluzan, R. and Levillain, R. (1966). *Nature, Lond.* **212,** 688–691.

Chambers, V. C. and Weiser, R. S. (1969). *Cancer Res.* **29,** 301–317.

Chang, Y. H. (1964). *J. nat. Cancer Inst.* **32,** 19–35.

Chang, Y. H. (1969). *Expl. Cell Res.* **54,** 42–48.

Chapman, J. A., Elves, M. W. and Gough, J. (1967a). *J. cell. Sci.* **2,** 359–370.

Chapman, J. A., Gough, J. and Elves, M. W. (1967b). *J. cell. Sci.* **2,** 371–376.

Christensen, R. G. and Marshall, J. M. (1965). *J. Cell Biol.* **25,** 443–457.

Clark, S. L. (1962). *Am. J. Anat.* **110,** 217–258.

Clark, S. L. (1963). *Am. J. Anat.* **112,** 1–34.

Clark, S. L. (1968). *J. exp. Med.* **128,** 927–957.

Clegg, E. J. and Macmillan, E. W. (1965). *J. Anat.* **99,** 219–229.

Cliff, W. J. (1963). *Phil. Trans. Roy. Soc. B.* **246,** 305–325.

Cline, N. S. and Lehrer, R. I. (1968). *Blood* **32,** 423–435.

Cline, M. J. and Swett, V. C. (1968). *J. exp. Med.* **128,** 1309–1324.

Cohen, A. S. (1964). *J. Ultrastruct. Res.* **10**, 124–144.

Cohen, A. S. (1965). *Int. Rev. exp. Path.* **4**, 159–243.

Cohen, S., Vassalli, P., McCluskey, R. T. and Benacerraf, B. (1966). *Lab. Invest.* **15**, 1143–1155.

Cohn, Z. A. (1963a). *J. exp. Med.* **117**, 27–42.

Cohn, Z. A. (1963b). *J. exp. Med.* **117**, 43–53.

Cohn, Z. A. (1966). *J. exp. Med.* **124**, 557–571.

Cohn, Z. A. (1968). *Adv. Immunol.* **9**, 163–214.

Cohn Z. A. (1970). *In* "The Mononuclear Phagocytes" (van Furth, R. ed.), Blackwell, London.

Cohn, Z. A. and Benson, B. (1965a). *J. exp. Med.* **121**, 153–169.

Cohn, Z. A. and Benson, B. (1965b). *J. exp. Med.* **121**, 835–848.

Cohn, Z. A. and Benson, B. (1965c). *J. exp. Med.* **122**, 455–466.

Cohn, Z. A. and Ehrenreich, B. A. (1969). *J. exp. Med.* **129**, 201–226.

Cohn, Z. A., Fedorko, M. E. and Hirsch, J. G. (1966a). *J. exp. Med.* **123**, 757–766.

Cohn, Z. A., Hirsch, J. G. and Fedorko, M. E. (1966b). *J. exp. Med.* **123**, 747–756.

Cohn, Z. A. and Parks, E. (1967a). *J. exp. Med.* **125**, 213–230.

Cohn, Z. A. and Parks, E. (1967b). *J. exp. Med.* **125**, 1091–1104.

Cohn, Z. A. and Parks, E. (1967c). *J. exp. Med.* **125**, 417.

Cohn, Z. A. and Weiner, E. (1963a). *J. exp. Med.* **118**, 991–1008.

Cohn, Z. A. and Weiner, E. (1963b). *J. exp. Med.* **118**, 1009–1021.

Collet, A. J. (1970). *Anat. Rec.* **167**, 277–289.

Collet, A. J. and Petrik, P. (1971a). *Z. Zellforsch. Mikrosk. Anat.* **116**, 464–476.

Collet, A. J. and Petrik, P. (1971b). *Z. Zellforsch. Mikrosk. Anat.* **116**, 477–486.

Colwell, C. A. and Hess, A. R. (1963). *Am. Rev. Resp. Dis.* **88**, 47–54.

Conalty, M. L. and Jackson, R. D. (1962). *Br. J. exp. Path.* **43**, 650–654.

Cookson, F. B. (1971). *Br. J. exp. Path.* **52**, 62–69.

Cooper, G. N. and Stuart, A. E. (1961). *Nature, Lond.* **191**, 294–295.

Cooper, G. N. and West, D. (1964). *Aust. J. exp. Biol. Med.* **40**, 485–498.

Corrin, B., Clark, A. E. and Spencer, H. (1969). *J. Anat., Lond.* **104**, 65–70.

Cotran, R. (1965). *Exp. Mol. Path.* **4**, 217–231.

Cowan, W. K. and Sorenson, G. D. (1964). *Lab. Invest.* **13**, 353–370.

Crosby, W. H. (1959). *Blood* **14**, 399–408.

Curran, R. C. and Clark, A. E. (1964). *J. Path. Bact.* **88**, 489–502.

Curran, R. C., Lovell, D. and Clark, A. E. (1966). *J. Path. Bact.* **91**, 429–439.

Daems, W. Th. and Persijn, J. P. (1964). *In* "Electron Microscopy" (Titbach, M. ed.), pp. 225–226, Czech. Acad. Sci., Prague.

Dannenberg, A. M. (1968). *Bact. Rev.* **32**, 85–102.

Dannenberg, A. M. and Bennett, W. E. (1964). *J. cell. Biol.* **21**, 1–13.

Dannenberg, A. M., Burstone, M. S., Walter, P. C. and Kinsley, J. W. (1963a). *J. Cell Biol.* **17**, 465–486.

Dannenberg, A. M., Kapral, F. A. and Walter, P. C. (1963b). *J. Immunol.* **90**, 448–465.

Davey, M. J. and Asherson, G. L. (1967). *Immunology* **12**, 13–20.

David, J. R. (1968a). *Fedn. Proc. Fedn. Am. Socs exp. Biol.* **27,** 6–12.

David, J. R. (1968b). *Cancer Res.* **28,** 1287–1291.

David, J. R., Al Askari, S., Lawrence, H. S. and Thomas, L. (1964). *J. Immunol.* **93,** 264–273.

Davis, J. M. G. (1963a). *Br. J. exp. Path.* **44,** 454–464.

Davis, J. M. G. (1963b). *Br. J. exp. Path.* **44,** 568–575.

Davis, J. M. G. (1964). *Br. J. exp. Path.* **45,** 634–641.

Day, A. J. (1960). *Q. Jl exp. Physiol.* **45,** 220–228.

Day, A. J. (1964). *J. Atheroscler. Res.* **4,** 117–130.

Day, A. J. and French, J. E. (1959). *Q. Jl exp. Physiol.* **44,** 239–243.

Day, A. J. and French, J. E. (1961). *J. Path. Bact.* **81,** 247–248.

Day, A. J. and Harris, P. M. (1960). *Q. Jl exp. Physiol.* **45,** 213–219.

Deane, H. W. (1964). *Anat. Rec.* **149,** 453–473.

de Haan, J. and Hoekstra, R. A. (1927). *Arch. exp. Zellforsch* **5,** 35–45.

Deno, R. A. (1936). *Am. J. Anat.* **60,** 433–471.

De Petris, S., Karlsbad, G. and Pernis, B. (1962). *J. Ultrastruct. Res.* **7,** 39–55.

Despont, J. P. and Cruchaud, A. (1969). *Nature, Lond.* **223,** 838–839.

Diluzio, N. R., Salky, N. K., Riggi, S. J. and Ladman, A. J. (1964). *Proc. Jap. Soc. Res.* **4,** 15–30.

Dorfman, R. F. (1961). *Nature, Lond.* **190,** 1021–1022.

Doty, P. (1968). *In* "Lysosomes in Biology and Pathology" (Dingle, J. T. & Fell, H. B., eds), North Holland, Amsterdam.

Dougherty, T. F. (1944). *Am. J. Anat.* **74,** 61–96.

Downey, R. J. and Diedrich, B. F. (1968). *Expl. Cell Res.* **50,** 483–489.

Drinker, C. K. and Yoffey, J. M. (1941). "Lymphatics, Lymph and Lymphoid tissue". Cambridge University Press, London.

Duff, G. L., McMillan, G. C. and Lautsch, E. V. (1954). *Am. J. Path.* **30,** 941–955.

Duff, G. L., McMillan, G. C. and Ritchie, A. C. (1957). *Am. J. Path.* **33,** 845–874.

Duguid, J. B. (1946). *J. Path. Bact.* **58,** 207–212.

Dumonde, D. C., Wolstencroft, R. A., Panayi, G. S., Matthew, M., Morley, J. and Howson, W. T. (1969). *Nature, Lond.* **224,** 38–42.

Dumont, A. (1969). *J. Ultrastruct. Res.* **29,** 191–209.

Dumont, A. and Robert, A. (1970). *Lab. Invest.* **23,** 278–286.

Dumont, A. and Sheldon, H. (1965). *Lab. Invest.* **14,** 2034–2055.

Dumont, A. E., Stertzer, S. M. and Mulholland, J. H. (1962). *Am. J. Physiol.* **202,** 704–706.

Dunning, H. S. and Furth, J. (1935). *Am. J. Path.* **11,** 895–913.

Dunning, H. S. and Stevenson, L. (1934). *Am. J. Path.* **10,** 343–348.

Ebert, R. H. and Florey, H. W. (1939). *Br. J. exp. Path.* **20,** 342–356.

Edwards, V. D. and Simon, S. T. (1970). *J. Ultrastruct. Res.* **33,** 187–201.

Ehrenreich, B. A. and Cohn, Z. A. (1968). *J. Cell Biol.* **38,** 244–248.

Ehrenreich, B. A. and Cohn, Z. A. (1969). *J. exp. Med.* **129,** 227–243.

Ehrenstein, G. and Lockner, D. (1958). *Nature, Lond.* **181,** 911.

Elias, P. M. and Epstein, W. L. (1968). *Am. J. Path.* **52,** 1207–1223.
Enders, A. C. and King, B. F. (1970). *Anat. Rec.* **167,** 231–251.
Enzinger, F. M. (1970). *Cancer, N.Y.* **26,** 1029–1041.
Epstein, W. L. (1967). *Prog. Allergy* **11,** 36–88.
Epstein, W. L., Skahen, J. R. and Krasnobrod, H. (1963). *Am. J. Path.* **43,** 391–405.
Eskeland, G. (1967). "Regeneration of Peritoneum; An Experimental Study". Universitets forlaget (Oslo). *Acta Pathol. Microbiol. Scand.* (1966). **68,** 355–378, 379–395, 501–516.
Essner, E. (1960). *J. biophys. biochem. Cytol.* **7,** 329–334.
Evans, R. and Alexander, P. (1970). *Nature, Lond.* **228,** 620–622.

Fahimi, H. D. (1970). *J. cell. Biol.* **47,** 247–262.
Farquar, M. A. and Hartmann, J. F. (1967). *J. Neuropath. exp. Neurol.* **16,** 18–39.
Fauve, R. M. and Dekaris, D. (1968). *Science, N.Y.* **160,** 795–796.
Fedorko, M. E., Hirsch, J. G. and Cohn, Z. A. (1968a). *J. Cell Biol.* **38,** 377–391.
Fedorko, M. E., Hirsch, J. G. and Cohn, Z. A. (1968b). *J. Cell Biol.* **38,** 392–402.
Felix, M. D. and Dalton, A. J. (1956). *J. biophys. biochem. Cytol.* **2,** Suppl. 109–114.
Fenn, W. (1921). *J. gen. Physiol.* **4,** 373–385.
Field, E. J. (1957). *J. Neuropath. exp. Neurol.* **16,** 48–56.
Fischer, R. (1970). *In* "The Mononuclear Phagocyte" (van Furth, R. ed.), Blackwell, London.
Fischman, D. A. and Hay, E. D. (1962). *Anat. Rec.* **143,** 329–334.
Fishman, M. (1961). *J. exp. Med.* **114,** 837–856.
Fishman, M. and Adler, F. L. (1963). *J. exp. Med.* **117,** 595–602.
Foot, N. (1925). *Anat. Rec.* **30,** 15–51.
Forbes, I. J. and Mackaness, G. B. (1963). *Lancet* **ii,** 1203–1204.
Fox, H. (1967). *J. Path. Bact.* **93,** 710–717.
Fox, H. and Kharkongor, F. N. (1970). *J. Path. Bact.* **101,** 267–276.
French, J. E. and Morris, B. (1960). *J. Path. Bact.* **79,** 11.
Fresen, O. and Wellensiek, H. J. (1959). *Verh. dtsch. Ges. Pathol.* **42,** 353–363.
Friend, D. S. and Farquar, M. G. (1967). *J. Cell Biol.* **35,** 357–376.
Friend, D. S., Rosenau, W., Winfield, J. S. and Moon, H. D. (1969). *Lab. Invest.* **20,** 275–282.

Gabrieli, E. R., Pyzikiewicz, T. and Mlodozeniec, P. (1967). *J. reticuloendothel. Soc.* **4,** 223–227.
Gad, B. and Clark, S. L., Jr. (1968). *Am. J. Anat.* **122,** 573–606.
Galindo, B. and Imaeda, T. (1962). *Anat. Rec.* **143,** 399–405.
Galindo, B. and Imaeda, T. (1966). *Lab. Invest.* **15,** 1659–1681.
Galindo, B. Imaeda, T. and Kanetsuna, F. (1969). *J. reticuloendothel. Soc.* **6,** 59–77.
Gall, E. A. (1958). *Ann. N.Y. Acad. Sci.* **73,** 120–130.
Gazayerli, M. el. (1936). *J. Path. Bact.* **43,** 357–366.
Gedigk, P. and Bontke, E. (1957). *Virchows Arch.* **330,** 538–568.
Geer, J. C. (1965). *Am. J. Path.* **47,** 241–252.

Geer, J. C., McGill, H. C. and Strong, J. P. (1961). *Am. J. Path.* **38**, 263–288.

George, M. and Vaughan, J. H. (1962). *Proc. Soc. exp. Biol.* **111**, 514–521.

Gershon, R. K. and Carter, R. L. (1967a). *Am. J. Path.* **50**, 137–157.

Gershon, R. K., Carter, R. L. and Lane, N. J. (1967b). *Am. J. Path.* **51**, 1111–1134.

Gershon, R. K. and Carter, R. L. (1970). *Nature, Lond.* **226**, 368–370.

Gershon, Z. and Olitski, A. L. (1965). *Proc. Soc. exp. Biol.* **119**, 32–34.

Ghani, A. R. (1969). *J. Path.* **97**, 11–21.

Gieseking, R. (1963). *Beitr. Path. Anat.* **128**, 259–282.

Gillman, J., Gillman, T. and Gilbert, C. (1949). *S. Afr. J. med. Sci.* **14**, 21–83.

Gillman, T. and Wright, L. J. (1966). *Nature, Lond.* **209**, 263–265.

Glasgow, L. A. (1965). *J. exp. Med.* **121**, 1001–1018.

Glasgow, L. A. (1966). *J. Bact.* **91**, 2185–2191.

Glees, P. (1955). "Neuroglia Morphology and Function". Blackwell, Oxford.

Goggins, J. F., Lazarus, G. S. and Fullmer, H. M. (1968). *J. Histochem. Cytochem.* **16**, 688–692.

Goldberg, B., Kantor, F. S. and Benacerraf, B. (1962). *Br. J. exp. Path.* **43**, 621–626.

Goldfischer, S., Novikoff, A. B., Albala, A. and Biempica, L. (1970). *J. Cell Biol.* **44**, 513–530.

Goldman, A. S. and Walker, B. E. (1963). *Lab. Invest.* **11**, 808–813.

Goldstein, M. N. (1954). *Anat. Rec.* **118**, 577–592.

Goldstein, M. N. and McCormick, T. (1957). *Am. J. Path.* **33**, 737–747.

Gomori, G. (1941). *Archs Path.* **32**, 189–199.

Gonatas, N. K., Zimmerman, H. M. and Levine, S. (1963). *Am. J. Path.* **42**, 455–469.

Gonatas, N. K., Levine, S. and Shoulson, R. (1964). *Am. J. Path.* **44**, 565–583.

Gonzales, F. and Karnovsky, M. J. (1961). *J. biophys. biochem. Cytol.* **9**, 299–316.

Goodman, J. W. (1964). *Blood* **23**, 18–26.

Gordon, G. B. and King, D. W. (1960). *Am. J. Path.* **37**, 279–291.

Gottlieb, A. A., Glisik, V. R. and Doty, P. (1967). *Proc. natn. Acad. Sci., U.S.A.* **57**, 1849–1856.

Grampa, G. (1971). "Pathology Annual", pp. 147–169 (Sommers, S. C., ed.), Butterworths, London.

Granger, G. A. and Weiser, R. S. (1964). *Science, N.Y.* **145**, 1427–1429.

Grogg, E. and Pearse, A. G. E. (1952). *Br. J. exp. Path.* **33**, 567–576.

Gusek, W. (1959). *Symp. Ital. Ges. Pathol.* 35–63, Instituto per la diffusione di opere scientifiche. Milan.

Gusek, W. (1964). *Med. Welt.* 850–866.

Gusek, W. and Naumann, P. (1959). *Verh. dtsch. Ges. Path.* **43**, 254–257.

Hahn, H. H., Char, D. C., Postel, W. B. and Wood, W. B. (1967). *J. exp. Med.* **126**, 385–394.

Hall, J. G., Morris, B. M., Moreno, G. D. and Bessis, M. (1967). *J. exp. Med.* **125**, 91–110.

Hampton, J. C. (1964). *In* "Electron Microscope Anatomy" (Kurtz, S. M., ed.), pp. 41–58. Academic Press, New York and London.

H

Hampton, J. C. (1958). *Acta. Anat.* **32,** 262–291.

Han, S. S. and Avery, J. K. (1965). *Anat. Rec.* **151,** 41–58.

Han, S. S., Han, I. H. and Johnson, A. G. (1970). *Am. J. Anat.* **129,** 141–168.

Hancox, N. M. (1956). *In* "The Biochemistry and Physiology of Bone", Academic Press, London and New York.

Hancox, N. M. and Boothroyd, B. (1961). *J. biophys. biochem. Cytol.* **3,** 651–661.

Hanna, M. G. and Szakal, A. K. (1968). *J. Immunol.* **101,** 949–962.

Hard, G. C. (1969). *Lab. Invest.* **29,** 309–315.

Hard, G. C. (1970). *Br. J. exp. Path.* **51,** 97–105.

Harris, H. (1953). *Br. J. exp. Path.* **34,** 276–279.

Harris, H. (1954). *Physiol. Rev.* **34,** 529–562.

Hart, P. d'A. (1968). *Science, N.Y.* **162,** 686–689.

Hashimoto, M. (1966). *Tohoku J. exp. Med.* **89,** 177–191.

Hatasa, K. and Nakamura, T. (1965). *Z. Zellforsch. Mikrosk. Anat.* **68,** 266–277.

Hayashi, M. and Fishman, W. H. (1962). *J. Histochem. Cytochem.* **10,** 101–108.

Heise, E. R. and Myrvik, Q. N. (1967). *J. reticuloendothel. Soc.* **4,** 510–523.

Helminen, H. J. and Ericcson, J. L. E. (1968a). *J. Ultrastr. Res.* **25,** 214–227.

Helminen, H. J. and Ericcson, J. L. E. (1968b). *J. Ultrastr. Res.* **25,** 228–239.

Helminen, H. J., Ericcson, J. L. and Orrenius, S. (1968). *J. Ultrastr. Res.* **25,** 240–252.

Heppleston, A. G. and Styles, J. A. (1967). *Nature, Lond.* **214,** 521–522.

Herbeuval-Bolikowska, H., Fourot-Bauzon, M., Robert-Hettich, C. and Christophe, M. (1966). *Nouv. Rev. Fr. Hemat.* **6,** 576–583.

Herndon, R. M. (1964). *J. Cell Biol.* **23,** 277–293.

Hersh, E. M. and Harris, J. E. (1968). *J. Immunol.* **100,** 1184–1194.

Hess, M. W. and Luscher, E. F. (1970). *Expl. Cell Res.* **59,** 193–196.

Hess, R. and Staubli, W. (1963). *Am. J. Path.* **43,** 301–335.

Hirsch, G. C. (1965). *Ann. Rev. Microbiol.* **19,** 339–350.

Hirsch, G. C. and Fedorko, M. E. (1970). *In* "The Mononuclear Phagocytes" (van Furth, R., ed.). Blackwell, London.

Hirsch, J. G., Fedorko, M. E. and Cohn, Z. A. (1968). *J. Cell Biol.* **38,** 629–632.

Hofbauer, J. (1925). *Am. J. Obstet. Gynec.* **10,** 1.

Holt, P. F. and Young, D. K. (1967). *J. Path. Bact.* **93,** 696–698.

Holub, M. (1962). *Ann. N.Y. Acad. Sci.* **99,** 477–486.

Horn, R. G., Koenig, M. G., Goodman, J. S. and Collins, R. D. (1969). *Lab. Invest.* **21,** 406–414.

Horta, S.da. (1967). *Ann. N.Y. Acad. Sci.* **145,** 676–699.

Hortega, P. del. (1932). *In* "Cytology and Cellular Pathology of the Nervous System." Hoeber, New York.

Howard, J. G. (1959). *J. Path. Bact.* **78,** 465–470.

Howard, J. G. (1961). *Scot. med. J.* **6,** 60–82.

Howard, J. G. and Benacerraf, B. (1966). *Br. J. exp. Path.* **47,** 193–200.

Hudson, G. (1968). *Acta Anat.* **71,** 100–107.

Hudson, G. (1969). *Acta Anat.* **73,** 136–141.

Hudson, G. and Yoffey, J. M. (1963). *J. Anat.* **97,** 409–416.

Hudson, G. and Yoffey, J. M. (1968). *J. Anat.* **103,** 515–525.

Hughes-Jones, N. C. (1961a). *Clin. Sci.* **20**, 315–322.
Hughes-Jones, N. C. (1961b). *Clin. Sci.* **20**, 323–332.
Huhn, D. (1966). *Blut* **13**, 1–14.
Huhn, D. and Steidle, C. (1967). *Z. Zellforsch. Mikrosk. Anat.* **82**, 391–406.
Humphrey, J. H. (1969). *Antibiot. Chemother.* (*Basel*). **15**, 7–23.
Humphrey, J. H., Askonas, B. A., Auzins, I., Schechter, I. and Sela, M. (1967). *Immunology* **13**, 71–86.

Imaeda, T. (1960). *J. invest. Derm.* **34**, 331–337.
Irwin, D. A. (1932). *Can. med. Ass. J.* **27**, 353–356.
Ito, T. and Hoshino, T. (1962). *Z. Zellforsch. Mikrosk. Anat.* **56**, 445–464.
Ito, T. and Miura, M. (1966). *Proc. Jap. Soc. Res.* **6**, 127–140.

Jacoby, F. (1965). *In* "Cells and Tissues in Culture" (Willmer, E. N., ed.), Vol. 2, pp. 1–93. Academic Press, London and New York.
Jacques, P. J. (1970). *In* "Lysosomes in Biology and Pathology" (Dingle, J. T. and Fell, H. B., eds), Vol. 2, pp. 395–420. (1969). North Holland, Amsterdam.
Jaffe, R. H. (1938). *In* "Handbook of Hematology" (Downey, H., ed.), Vol. 2, pp. 975–1271. Hamilton, London.
Jayatilaka, A. J. (1965). *J. Anat. Lond.* **155**, 117–132.
Jee, W. S. S. and Nolan, P. D. (1963). *Nature, Lond.* **200**, 225–226.
Jenkin, C. and Benacerraf, B. (1960). *J. exp. Med.* **112**, 403–417.
Jennings, J. F. and Hughes, L. A. (1969). *Nature, Lond.* **221**, 79–80.
Jeunet, F. S., Cain, W. A. and Good, R. A. (1969). *J. reticuloendothel. Soc.* **6**, 391–410.
Jeunet, F. S. and Good, R. A. (1967). *J. reticuloendothel. Soc.* **4**, 351–369.
Johanovsky, J. (1960). *Immunology* **3**, 179–189.
Journey, L. J. (1963). *Cancer Res.* **24**, 1391–1436.
Journey, L. J. and Amos, D. B. (1962). *Cancer Res.* **22**, 998–1001.

Kajikawa, K. (1964). *Tohoku J. exp. Med.* **81**, 350–365.
Kajikawa, K., Nakanishi, I. and Kondo, K. (1970). *Recent Adv. RES.* **9**, 83–95.
Kallio, D. M., Garant, P. R. and Minkin, C. (1971). *J. Ultrastruct. Res.* **37**, 169–177.
Kallio, D. M., Garant, P. R. and Minkin, C. (1972). *J. Ultrastruct. Res.* **39**, 205–216.
Karlsbad, G., Kessel, R. W. I., de Petris, S. and Monaco, L. (1964). *J. gen. Microbiol.* **35**, 383–390.
Karnovsky, M. L. (1962). *Physiol. Rev.* **42**, 143–168.
Karrer, H. E. (1958). *J. biophys. biochem. Cytol.* **4**, 693–700.
Karrer, H. E. (1961). *J. Ultrastruct. Res.* **5**, 116–141.
Kawabata, S. and Asakawa, M. (1965). *Proc. Jap. Soc. Res.* **5**, 78–89.
Keene, W. R. and Jandl, J. M. (1965). *Blood* **26**, 157–175.
Keller, H. U. and Sorkin, E. (1967). *Int. Arch. Allergy* **31**, 575.
Keller, H. U. and Sorkin, E. (1968). *Experientia* **24**, 641.
Kelly, L. S. and Dobson, E. L. (1971). *Br. J. exp. Path.* **52**, 88–99.
Kelly, L. S., Brown, B. A. and Dobson, E. L. (1962). *Proc. Soc. exp. Biol. Med.* **110**, 555–559.

Khoo, K. K. and Mackaness, G. B. (1964). *Aust. J. exp. Biol. med. Sci.* **42**, 707–716.
Kinsky, R. G., Christie, G. H., Elson, J. and Howard, J. G. (1969). *Br. J. exp. Path.* **50**, 438–447.
Kirkpatrick, J. B. (1967). *Am. J. Path.* **50**, 291–309.
Kirkpatrick, J. B. and Sorenson, G. D. (1965). *Exp. molec. Path.* **4**, 627–639.
Kiyono, K. (1914). "Die Vitale Carminspeicherung", Fischer Verlag, Jena.
Klaus, M., Reiss, O. K., Tooley, W. H., Piel, C. and Clements, J. A. (1962). *Science, N.Y.* **137**, 750–751.
Klemperer, P. (1938). *In* "Handbook of Hematology" (Downey, H. ed.), Vol. 3, pp. 1591–1754. Hoeber, New York.
Kolliker, A. (1873). "Die normale Resorption des Knochengewebes", Vogel, Leipzig.
Kolouth, F. (1939). *Am. J. Path.* **15**, 413–428.
Kolsch, E. and Mitchison, N. A. (1969). *J. exp. Med.* **128**, 1059–1079.
Konigsmark, B. W. and Sidman, R. L. (1963). *J. Neuropath. exp. Neurol.* **22**, 643–676.
Kono, Y. and Ho, M. (1965). *Virology* **25**, 164–166.
Korn, E. D. and Weisman, R. A. (1967). *J. Cell Biol.* **34**, 219–227.
Kosunen, T. V., Waksman, B. H., Flax, M. H. and Tihen, W. S. (1963a). *Immunology* **6**, 276–290.
Kosunen, T. V., Waksman, B. H. and Samuelson, I. K. (1963b). *J. Neuropath. exp. Neurol.* **22**, 367–380.
Koyama, S., Sadako, A. and Depuchi, K. (1964). *Mie med. J.* **14**, 143–188.
Koyhani, E. and Bessis, M. (1969). *Nouv. Rev. Fr. Hemat.* **9**, 803–816.
Kubie, L. S. (1927). *J. exp. Med.* **46**, 615–626.
Kuhn, N. O. and Olivier, M. I. (1965). *J. Cell Biol.* **26**, 977–979.

Lawson, N. S., Schintzer, B. and Smith, E. B. (1969). *Archs Path.* **87**, 491–501.
Lay, W. H. and Nussenzweig, V. (1968). *J. exp. Med.* **128**, 991–1007.
Lay, W. H. and Nussenzweig, V. (1969). *J. Immunol.* **102**, 1172–1178.
Leake, E. S. and Heise, E. R. (1967). "The Reticuloendothelial System and Atherosclerosis", pp. 136–149.
Leake, E. S. and Myrvik, Q. N. (1966). *J. reticuloendothel. Soc.* **3**, 83–100.
Leake, E. S. and Myrvik, Q. N. (1968). *J. reticuloendothel. Soc.* **5**, 33–53.
Leake, E. S. and Myrvik, Q. N. (1970). *J. reticuloendothel. Soc.* **8**, 407–420.
Leake, E. S., Evans, D. G. and Myrvik, Q. N. (1971). *J. reticuloendothel. Soc.* **9**, 174–199.
Leary, T. (1941). *Archs Path.* **32**, 507–555.
Leary, T. (1949). *Archs Path.* **47**, 1–36.
Lewis, O. J. (1961). *J. Anat., Lond.* **91**, 245–250.
Lewis, W. H. (1924). *Bull. Johns Hopk. Hosp.* **35**, 183–185.
Lewis, W. H. (1931). *Bull. Johns Hopk. Hosp.* **49**, 17.
Lewis, W. H. and Gey, G. O. (1923). *Bull. Johns Hopk. Hosp.* **34**, 369–371.
Lewis, M. G. Ikonopisov, R. L., Nairn, R. C., Phillips, T. M., Fairley, G. H., Bodenham, D. C. and Alexander, P. (1969). *Br. med. J.* **3**, 547–552.
Lewis, W. H. and Webster, L. T. (1921). *J. exp. Med.* **33**, 261.

Lind, P. E. (1968). *Aust. J. exp. Biol. med. Sci.* **46,** 189–208.

Lindblad, G. and Bjorkman, N. (1964). *Acta. Path. Microbiol. Scand.* **62,** 155–164.

Lison, L. and Smulders, J. (1948). *Nature, Lond.* **162,** 65.

Lobel, B. L. and Deane, H. W. (1962). *Endocrinology* **70,** 567–578.

LoBuglio, A. F., Cotran, R. S. and Jandl, J. H. (1967). *Science, N.Y.* **158,** 1582–1585.

Lockard, V. G., Sharbaugh, R. J., Arhelger, R. B. and Grogan, J. B. (1971). *J. reticuloendothel. Soc.* **9,** 97–107.

Lockwood, W. R. and Allison, F. (1966). *Br. J. exp. Path.* **47,** 158–162.

Low, F. N. (1952). *Anat. Rec.* **113,** 437–459.

Low, F. N. and Freeman, J. A. (1958). "Electron Microscopic Atlas of Normal and Leukaemic Blood". McGraw Hill, New York.

Low, F. N. and Sampaio, M. M. (1957). *Anat. Rec.* **127,** 51–56.

Lozzio, B. B. (1967). *J. reticuloendothel. Soc.* **4,** 85–108.

Luckett, W. P. (1970). *Anat. Rec.* **167,** 141–164.

Lurie, M. B. (1939). *J. exp. Med.* **69,** 579–606.

Luse, S. A. (1956). *J. biophys. biochem. Cytol.* **2,** 531–541.

Machado, E., Lozzio, B. B. and Royer, M. (1968). *J. reticuloendothel. Soc.* **5,** 297–314.

Mackaness, G. B. (1962). *J. exp. Med.* **116,** 381–406.

Mackaness, G. B. and Blanden, R. V. (1967). *Progr. Allergy* **11,** 89–140.

McCallum, D. K. (1969a). *J. reticuloendothel. Soc.* **6,** 232–252.

McCallum, D. K. (1969b). *J. reticuloendothel. Soc.* **6,** 253–270.

McCutcheon, M. (1946). *Physiol. Rev.* **26,** 319–336.

McDevitt, H., Askonas, B. A., Humphrey, J. H., Schechter, I. and Sela, M. (1966). *Immunology* **11,** 337–351.

MacDonald, R., MacSween, R. N. M. and Pechest, G. S. (1969). *Lab. Invest.* **21,** 236–245.

McFadden, K. D. (1968). *J. reticuloendothel. Soc.* **5,** 385–398.

Mackenzie, D. H. (1971). *Br. J. Cancer,* **25,** 458–461.

MacLaurin, B. P. (1969). *Aust. J. exp. Biol. med. Sci.* **47,** 105–112.

Majno, G. and Palade, G. E. (1961). *J. Biophys. biochem. Cytol.* **11,** 571–605.

Majno, G. (1964). *In* "Handbook of Physiology", Sect. 2, Vol. 3, pp. 2293–2375. Am. Physiol. Soc.

De Man, J. C. H. (1968). *J. Path. Bact.* **95,** 123–126.

Mandel, T., Byrt, P. and Ada, G. L. (1969). *Exp. Cell Res.* **58,** 175–182.

Marchand, F. (1924). *Haematologica* **5,** 304.

Marshall, A. H. E. (1946). *J. Path. Bact.* **58,** 729–738.

Marshall, A. H. E. (1956). "An Outline of the Cytology and Pathology of the Reticular Tissue". Oliver and Boyd.

Marshall, A. H. E. and White, R. G. (1950). *Brit. J. exp. Path.* **31,** 157–174.

Maruyama, K. and Masuda, T. (1965). *Ann. Rep. Virus Inst. Kyoto.* **88,** 50–61.

MacSween, R. N. M. and MacDonald, R. A. (1969). *Lab. Invest.* **21,** 230–235.

Matter, A., Orci, L., Fossman, W. G. and Rouiller, Ch. (1968). *J. Ultrastruct. Res.* **23,** 272–279.

Maximow, A. A. (1928). *In* "Special Cytology" (Cowdry, E. V., ed.), pp. 711–770.

Maximow, A. A. and Bloom, W. (1931). "A Textbook of Histology". Saunders, Philadelphia and London.

Mayberry, H. E. (1964). *Anat. Rec.* **149,** 99.

Mayhew, T. and Williams, M. A. (1971). *J. Anat., London.* **108,** 602.

Medawar, J. (1940). *Br. J. exp. Path.* **21,** 205–211.

Menzies, D. W. (1965). *Nature, Lond.* **208,** 163–165.

Merkow, L. P., Epstein, M., Sidransky, H., Verney, E. and Pardo, M. (1971). *Am. J. Path.* **62,** 57–66.

Merkow, L. P., Frich, J. C., Stifkin, M., Kyreages, C. G. and Pardo, M. (1971). *Cancer* **28,** 372–383.

Metcalf, D. and Ishidate, M. (1961). *Nature, Lond.* **191,** 305.

Metchnikoff, E. (1891). "Lectures on the Comparative Pathology of Inflammation". Reprinted 1968. Dove Publications, New York.

Metzger, G. V. and Casarett, L. J. (1969). *J. reticuloendothel. Soc.* **6,** 435–447.

Meyer, O. T., Dannenberg, A. M. and Mizunoe, K. (1970). *J. reticuloendothel. Soc.* **7,** 15–31.

Miescher, P. (1956). *In* "Physiopathology of the Reticuloendothelial System" (Halpern, B. N., Benacerraf, B. & Delafresnaye, J. F., eds), p. 147. Thomas, Springfield.

Milanesi, S. (1965a). *Boll. Soc. Ital. Biol. Sper.* **41,** 1221–1223.

Milanesi, S. (1965b). *Boll. Soc. Ital. Biol. Sper.* **41,** 1223–1225.

Mills, D. M. and Zucker-Franklin, D. (1969). *Am. J. Path.* **54,** 147–166.

Mims, C. A. (1964a). *Br. J. exp. Path.* **45,** 37–43.

Mims, C. A. (1964b). *Bact. Rev.* **28,** 30–71.

Moe, R. E. (1963). *Am. J. Anat.* **112,** 311–335.

Moe, R. E. (1964). *Am. J. Anat.* **114,** 341–370.

Monis, B., Weinberg, T. and Spector, G. J. (1968). *Br. J. exp. Path.* **49,** 302–310.

Moore, R. D. and Schoenberg, M. D. (1964a). *Am. J. Path.* **45,** 991–1006.

Moore, R. D. and Schoenberg, M. D. (1964b). *Br. J. exp. Path.* **45,** 488–497.

Moore, R. D., Mumaw, V. R. and Schoenberg, M. D. (1964). *Exp. molec. Path.* **3,** 31–50.

Morales, A. R., Fine, G., Horn, R. C. and Watson, J. H. C. (1969). *Lab. Invest.* **20,** 412–423.

Mori, M., Ishii, Y. and Onoe, T. (1969). *J. reticuloendothel. Soc.* **6,** 140–157.

Mori, M., Ishii, Y. and Onoe, T. (1971). *Z. Zellforsch. Mikrosk. Anat.* **112,** 158–172.

Mori, S. (1966). *Sapporo Igaku Zashi* **30,** 65–84.

Mori, S. and Leblond, C. P. (1969). *J. comp. Neurol.* **135,** 57–59.

Mori, Y. and Lennert, K. (1969). "Electron Microscopic Atlas of Lymph node Cytology and Pathology". Springer-Verlag, Heidelberg.

Morita, T. and Perkins, E. H. (1965). *J. reticuloendothel. Soc.* **2,** 406–419.

Mudd, S., McCutcheon, M. and Lucke, B. (1934). *Physiol. Rev.* **14,** 210–275.

Muir, A. R. and Golberg, L. (1961a). *Q. Jl exp. Physiol.* **46,** 289–298.

Muir, A. R. and Golberg, L. (1961b). *J. Path. Bact.* **82**, 471–482.

Myrvik, Q. N. and Heise, R. S. (1951). *Am. Rev. Tuberc.* **64**, 669–681.

Myrvik, Q. N., Leake, E. S. and Fariss, B. (1961a). *J. Immunol.* **86**, 128–132.

Myrvik, Q. N., Leake, E. S. and Fariss, B. (1961b). *J. Immunol.* **86**, 133–138.

Myrvik, Q. N., Leake, E. S. and Oshima, S. (1962). *J. Immunol.* **89**, 745–751.

Nabors, C. J., Berliner, D. L. and Dougherty, T. F. (1967). *J. reticuloendothel. Soc.* **4**, 237–253.

Nagano, Y., Kojima, Y., Arakawa, J. and Kanashiro, R. S. (1966). *Jap. J. exp. Med.* **36**, 481–487.

Nelson, D. (1969). "The Macrophage in Immunology". North Holland, Amsterdam.

Nicol, T. (1932). *J. Anat.* **66**, 181.

Nicol, T. (1935). *Trans. roy. Soc. Edinb.* **58**, 449.

Nicol, T. and Bilbey, D. L. J. (1958). *Nature, Lond.* **182**, 192.

Nicolescu, P. and Rouiller, Ch. (1967). *Z. Zellforsch. Mikrosk. Anat.* **76**, 313–338.

Nichols, B. A., Bainton, D. F. and Farquar, M. G. (1971). *J. Cell Biol.* **50**, 498–515.

Niemi, M., Harkoven, H. and Kokko, A. (1962). *J. Histochem. Cytochem.* **10**, 186–193.

Niemi, M. and Kormano, H. (1965). *Anat. Rec.* **151**, 159–170.

North, R. J. (1966a). *J. Ultrastruct. Res.* **16**, 83–95.

North, R. J. (1966b). *J. Ultrastruct. Res.* **16**, 96–108.

North, R. J. (1969a). *J. exp. Med.* **130**, 299–314.

North, R. J. (1969b). *J. exp. Med.* **130**, 315–326.

North, R. J. (1970a). *J. exp. Med.* **132**, 521–534.

North, R. J. (1970b). *J. exp. Med.* **132**, 535–545.

North, R. J. and Mackaness, G. B. (1963a). *Br. J. exp. Path.* **44**, 601–607.

North, R. J. and Machaness, G. B. (1963b). *Br. J. exp. Path.* **44**, 608–611.

Nossal, G. J. V., Abbot, A. and Mitchell, J. (1968a). *J. exp. Med.* **127**, 263–276.

Nossal, G. J. V., Abbot, A., Mitchell, J. and Lummus, Z. (1968b). *J. exp. Med.* **127**, 277–289.

Nossal, G. J. V., Ada, G. L. and Austin, C. M. (1964). *Aust. J. exp. Biol. med. Sci.* **42**, 311–330.

Nossall, G. J. V., Ada, G. L., Austin, C. M. and Pye, J. (1965). *Immunology* **9**, 349–357.

Novikoff, A. B. and Essner, E. (1960). *Am. J. Med.* **29**, 102–131.

Noyes, W. D., Bothwell, T. H. and Finch, C. A. (1960). *Br. J. Haemat.* **6**, 43–55.

Odor, D. C. (1956). *J. biophys. biochem. Cytol.* **2**, Supp. 105–108.

Oldfield, F. E. (1963). *Exp. Cell Res.* **30**, 125–138.

Onoe, T. and Tsukada, H. (1964). *Tohoku J. exp. Med.* **81**, 340–349.

Orci, L., Pictet, R. and Rouiller, C. (1967). *J. Microscopie* **6**, 413–417.

Oren, R., Farnham, A. E., Saito, K., Milofsky, E. and Karnovsky, M. L. (1963). *J. Cell Biol.* **17**, 487–502.

Orlic, D., Gordon, A. S. and Rhodin, J. A. G. (1965). *J. Ultrastruct. Res.* **13,** 516–542.

Ossermann, E. T. and Lawler, D. P. (1966). *J. exp. Med.* **124,** 921–952.

Palumbi, G. and Millonig, G. (1960). *Arch. ital. Anat. Embriol.* **65,** 155–167.

Panijel, J. and Cayeux, P. (1968). *Immunology* **14,** 769–780.

Papadimitriou, J. M. and Spector, W. G. (1971). *J. Path.* **105,** 187–204.

Papadimitriou, J. M. and Walters, M. N-I. (1968). *Am. J. Anat.* **123,** 475–488.

Parakkal, P. F. (1969a). *J. Ultrastruct. Res.* **29,** 210–217.

Parakkal, P. F. (1969b). *J. Cell Biol.* **41,** 345–354.

Parker, F. (1960). *Am. J. Path.* **36,** 19–53.

Parker, F. and Odland, G. F. (1966a). *Am. J. Path.* **48,** 197–239.

Parker, F. and Odland, G. F. (1966b). *Am. J. Path.* **48,** 451–482.

Parker, F. and Odland, G. F. (1969). *J. invest. Derm.* **52,** 136–147.

Parks, H. F. and Chiquoine, A. D. (1957). *In* "Electron Microscopy" (Rhodin, J. & Sjostrand, F. S., eds), pp. 151–154. Almqvist and Wiksell, Stockholm.

Patek, P. R., de Mignard, V. A. and Bernick, S. (1967). *J. reticuloendothel. Soc.* **4,** 211–218.

Paz, R. A. and Spector, W. G. (1962). *J. Path. Bact.* **84,** 85–103.

Pearsall, N. N. and Weiser, R. S. (1968a). *J. reticuloendothel. Soc.* **5,** 107–120.

Pearsall, N. N. and Weiser, R. S. (1968b). *J. reticuloendothel. Soc.* **5,** 121–133.

Pease, D. C. (1956). *Blood* **11,** 501–526.

Penfield, W. (1925). *Am. J. Path.* **1,** 77–90.

Perkins, E. H. and Makinodan, T. (1965). *J. Immunol.* **94,** 765–777.

Perkins, E. H., Nettesheim, P. and Morita, T. (1966). *J. reticuloendothel. Soc.* **3,** 71–82.

Perkins, E. H., Nettesheim, P., Morita, T. and Walberg, H. E. (1967). *In* "The Reticuloendothelial System in Atherosclerosis" (Diluzio, N. R. & Paoletti, R., eds), Plenum Press, New York.

Pernis, B., Bairati, A. and Milanesi, S. (1966). *Path. Microbiol. (Basel)* **29,** 837–853.

Petterson, J. C. (1964). *Anat. Rec.* **149,** 269–278.

Phillips, M. E. and Thorbecke, G. T. (1966). *Int. Arch. Allergy* **29,** 553–567.

Pictet, R., Orci, L., Forssmann, W. G. and Girardier, L. (1969a). *Z. Zellforsch. Mikrosk. Anat.* **96,** 372–399.

Pictet, R., Orci, L., Forssmann, W. G. and Girardier, L. (1969b). *Z. Zellforsch. Mikrosk. Anat.* **96,** 400–417.

Pincus, W. B. (1967). *J. reticuloendothel. Soc.* **4,** 140–150.

Pincus, W. B., Spanis, C. W. and Sintek, D. E. (1971). *J. reticuloendothel. Soc.* **9,** 552–567.

Pinkett, M. O., Cowdrey, C. R. and Nowell, P. C. (1966). *Am. J. Path.* **48,** 859–865.

Pisano, J. C. and Diluzio, N. R. (1970). *J. reticuloendothel. Soc.* **7,** 386–396.

Pisano, J. C., Diluzio, N. R. and Salky, N. K. (1970). *Nature, Lond.* **226,** 1049–1050.

Policard, A., Collet, A., Martin, J. C., Pregerman, S. and Reuet, C. (1963). *C. r. hebd. Séanc. Acad. Sci., Paris* **256**, 3404–3406.

Policard, A., Collet, A., Martin, J. C. and Reuet, C. (1965). *Z. Zellforsch. Mikrosk. Anat.* **66**, 96–105.

Pollock, E., Pegram, C. N. and Vasquez, J. J. (1971). *J. reticuloendothel. Soc.* **9**, 383–391.

Ponfick, E. (1869). *Virchows Arch. path. Anat.* **48**, 1–55.

Poole, J. C. F. and Florey, H. W. (1958). *J. Path. Bact.* **75**, 245–251.

Prose, P. H., Lee, L. and Balk, S. D. (1965). *Am. J. Path.* **47**, 403–417.

Rabinovitch, M. (1967a). *Expl. Cell Res.* **46**, 19–28.

Rabinovitch, M. (1967b). *J. Immunol.* **99**, 232–237.

Rabinovitch, M. (1967c). *J. Immunol.* **99**, 115–1120.

Rabinovitch, M. (1968). *Seminars Haematol.* **5**, 134–155.

Rabinovitch, M. (1970). *In* "The Mononuclear Phagocyte" (van Furth R., ed.), Blackwell, London.

Rabinovitch, M. and Gary, P. (1968). *Expl. Cell Res.* **52**, 363–369.

Rambourg, A. and Leblond, C. P. (1965). *J. Cell Biol.* **32**, 27–53.

Rannie, I. and Duguid, J. B. (1953). *J. Path. Bact.* **66**, 395–398.

Ranvier, L. (1870). *Arch. Physiol* **1**, 421–428.

Ranvier, L. (1890). *C. r. hebd. Séanc. Acad. Sci., Paris* **110**, 165.

Rappaport, H. (1966). "Tumours of the Hematopoietic System", Armed Forces Institute of Pathology, Washington, D.C.

Rebuck, J. W., Boyd, C. B. and Riddle, J. M. (1960). *Ann. N.Y. Acad. Sci.* **88**, 30–42.

Rebuck, J. W. and Crowley, J. H. (1955). *Ann. N.Y. Acad. Sci.* **59**, 757–794.

Renaut, J. (1907). *Arch. d'anat. microsc.* **9**, 495.

Resibois, A., Tondeur, M., Mockel, S. and Dustin, P. (1970). *Int. Rev. exp. Path.* **9**, 93–149.

Rhodes, J. M. and Lind, I. (1968). *Immunology* **14**, 511–525.

Rhodes, J. M., Lind, I., Birch-Andersen, A. and Ravn, H. (1970). *Immunology* **17**, 441–452.

Rich, A. R. and Lewis, M. R. (1932). *Bull. Johns Hopk. Hosp.* **50**, 115–119.

Richter, G. W. (1959). *J. exp. Med.* **109**, 197–216.

Rifkind, R. A. (1965). *Blood* **26**, 433–448.

Rifkind, R. A. (1966). *Am. J. Med.* **41**, 711–723.

Riggi, S. J. and Diluzio, N. R. (1961). *Am. J. Physiol.* **200**, 297–300.

Roberts, D. K. and Latta, J. S. (1964). *Anat. Rec.* **148**, 81–101.

Roberts, D. M., Themann, H., Knust, F. J., Preston, F. E. and Donaldson, J. R. (1970). *J. Path.* **100**, 249–255.

Robertson, J. S. (1952). *Aust. J. exp. Biol.* **30**, 59–71.

Robertson, W. F. (1900). *J. ment. Sci.* **46**, 733–752.

Roelants, G. E. and Goodman, J. W. (1969). *J. exp. Med.* **130**, 557–574.

Roser, B. (1965). *Aust. J. exp. Biol. med. Sci.* **43**, 553–562.

Roser, B. (1970). *J. reticuloendothel. Soc.* **8**, 139–161.

Roser, R. (1968). *J. reticuloendothel. Soc.* **5**, 455–471.

Ross, R. and Benditt, E. P. (1962). *J. Cell Biol.* **12,** 533–551.
Ross, R. and Odland, G. (1968). *J. Cell Biol.* **39,** 152–168.
Roth, S. L. and Porter, K. R. (1964). *J. Cell Biol.* **20,** 313–332.
Rouiller, Ch. and Jezequel, A. M. (1963). "The Liver", Vol. 1, pp. 195–265. Academic Press, New York and London.
Rous, P. (1925a). *J. exp. Med.* **41,** 379–397.
Rous, P. (1925b). *J. exp. Med.* **41,** 399–411.
Rous, P. and Beard, J. W. (1934). *J. exp. Med.* **59,** 577–591.
Rous, P. and Robertson, O. M. (1917). *J. exp. Med.* **25,** 651–664.
Russell, D. S. (1929). *Am. J. Path.* **5,** 451–458.
Russell, G. V. (1962). *Texas Rep. exp. Biol.* **20,** 338–351.
Russell, P. and Roser, B. (1966). *Aust. J. exp. Biol. med Sci.* **44,** 629–638.
Ryan, G. B. and Spector, W. G. (1969). *J. Path.* **99,** 139–151.
Ryan, G. B. and Spector, W. G. (1970). *Proc. roy. Soc. B.* **175,** 269–292.
Ryser, M. J. P. (1968). *Science, N.Y.* **159,** 390–396.

Sabin, F. R. (1939). *J. exp. Med.* **70,** 67–82.
Sagebiel, R. W. and Reed, T. H. (1968). *J. Cell Biol.* **36,** 595–602.
Saito, K. and Sutter, E. (1965). *J. exp. Med.* **121,** 727–738.
Sakuma, S. (1966). *Proc. Jap. Soc. Res.* **6,** 58–67.
Salvin, S. B. and Nishio, J. (1969). *J. Immunol.* **103,** 138–141.
Salvin, S. B., Sell, S. and Nishio, J. (1971). *J. Immunol.* **107,** 655–662.
Sanders, C. L. and Adee, R. R. (1969). *J. reticuloendothel. Soc.* **6,** 1–23.
Santos-Buch, C. A. and Treadwell, P. M. (1968). *Am. J. Path.* **51,** 505–525.
Saxl, P. and Donath, F. (1924). *Wien, Klin. Wchhschr.* **38,** 66–68.
Schmidt, F. C. (1960). *Anat. Anz.* **108,** 376–387.
Schneeberger-Keeley, E. E. and Burger, E. J., Jr. (1970). *Lab. Invest.* **22,** 361–369.
Schoenberg, M. D., Mumaw, V. R., Moore, R. D. and Weisberger, A. S. (1963). *Science, N.Y.* **143,** 964.
Schulz, R. L., Maynard, E. A. and Pease, D. C. (1957). *Am. J. Anat.* **100,** 369 408.
Schulz, H. (1959). "The Submicroscopic Anatomy and Pathology of the Lung", Springer, Berlin.
Schulz, P. (1965). *Arch. Exp. Veterinaermed.* **19,** 1341–1368.
Scott, B. L. (1967). *J. Ultrastruct. Res.* **19,** 417–431.
Scott, B. L. and Pease, D. C. (1956). *Anat. Rec.* **126,** 465–496.
Shands, J. W. (1967). *In* "Modern Trends in Immunology" (Cruickshank, R. & Wier, D. M., eds), Butterworths, London.
Shamoto, M. (1970). *Cancer,* **26,** 1102–1108.
Shirahama, T. and Cohen, A. S. (1970). *J. Ultrastruct. Res.* **33,** 587–597.
Shirahama, T., Cohen, A. S. and Rodger, O. G. (1971). *Expl. molec. Path.* **14,** 110–123.
Shorter, R. G. and Titus, J. L. (1962). *Proc. Staff Meet. Mayo Clinic.* **37,** 669–679.
Shorter, R. G., Titus, J. C. and Divertie, M. B. (1966). *Thorax* **21,** 32–37.
Simon, G. T. and Burke, J. S. (1970). *Am. J. Path.* **58,** 451–469.

Simon, G. and Pictet, R. (1964). *Acta Anat.* **57,** 163–171.

Simpson, M. E. (1922). *J. med. Res.* **43,** 78–144.

Singer, J. M., Adlersberg, L., Koenig, E. M., Ende, E. and Tchorsch, Y. (1969). *J. reticuloendothel. Soc.* **6,** 561–589.

Smith, E. B., White, D. C., Hartsock, R. J. and Dixon, A. C. (1967). *Am. J. Path.* **50,** 159–175.

Smith, C. W. and Goldman, A. S. (1970). *J. reticuloendothel. Soc.* **8,** 91–104.

Smith, J. B., Mackintosh, G. H. and Morris, B. (1970a). *J. Anat.* **107,** 87–100.

Smith, J. B., Mackintosh, G. H. and Morris, B. (1970b). *J. Path.* **100,** 21–30.

Smith, T. J. and Wagner, R. R. (1967a). *J. exp. Med.* **125,** 559–577.

Smith, T. J. and Wagner, R. R. (1967b). *J. exp. Med.* **125,** 579–593.

Snook, T. (1964). *Anat. Rec.* **148,** 129–160.

Solnitzky, T. (1937). *Anat. Rec.* **69,** 55–70.

Sorenson, G. D. (1960). *Am. J. Anat.* **107,** 73–96.

Sorenson, G. D., Heffner, W. A. and Kirkpatrick, J. B. (1964). *Am. J. Path.* **44,** 629–644.

Sorokin, S. (1966). *J. Histochem. Cytochem.* **14,** 884–897.

Spector, W. G., Walters, M. N. I. and Willoughby, D. A. (1965). *J. Path. Bact.* **90,** 181–192.

Spector, W. G. (1969). *Int. Rev. exp. Path.* **8,** 1–55.

Spector, W. G. and Coote, E. (1965). *J. Path. Bact.* **90,** 589–598.

Spector, W. G. and Lykke, A. W. J. (1966). *J. Path. Bact.* **92,** 163–177.

Spector, W. G. and Willoughby, D. A. (1963). *Bact. Rev.* **27,** 117–152.

Spector, W. G. and Willoughby, D. A. (1968). *J. Path. Bact.* **96,** 389–399.

Spector, W. G., Lykke, A. W. J. and Willoughby, D. A. (1967). *J. Path. Bact.* **93,** 101–107.

Spector, W. G., Heesom, N. and Stevens, J. E. (1968). *J. Path. Bact.* **96,** 203–213.

Spector, W. G., Reichhold, N. and Ryan, G. B. (1970). *J. Path.* **101,** 339–354.

Sprick, M. G. (1956). *Am. Rev. Tuberc.* **74,** 552–565.

Stastny, P. and Ziff, M. (1970). *J. reticuloendothel. Soc.* **7,** 140–146.

Steiner, J. W. (1961). *Am. J. Path.* **38,** 411–436.

Stevanovic, J., Webb, T. and Lapresle, C. I. (1962). *Ann. Inst. Pasteur* **103,** 276–284.

Stiffel, C., Mouton, D. and Biozzi, G. (1970). *In* "Mononuclear Phagocytes" (van Furth, R., ed.) Blackwell, London.

Still, W. J. S. and O'Neal, R. M. (1962). *Am. J. Path.* **48,** 197–239.

Straus, W. (1970). *J. Histochem. Cytochem.* **18,** 120–130.

Straus, W. (1970). *J. Histochem. Cytochem.* **18,** 131–142.

Stuart, A. E. (1962). *J. Path. Bact.* **84,** 193–200.

Stuart, A. E. (1967). *J. Path. Bact.* **93,** 338–340.

Stuart, A. E. (1970). "The Reticuloendothelial System", Livingstone, Edinburgh.

Stuart, A. E., Clark, J., Boulton, J. and Collee, J. G. (1969). *J. Path. Bact.* **97,** 93–98.

Stuart, A. E. and Davidson, A. E. (1971a). *J. Path.* **103,** 41–47.

Stuart, A. E. and Davidson, A. E. (1971b). *J. Path.* **103,** 194–198.

Stuart, A. E. and Davidson, A. E. (1971c). *J. Path.* **104**, 37–43.

Stuart, A. E., Biozzi, G., Stiffel, C., Halpern, B. N. and Moulon, D. (1960). *Br. J. exp. Path.* **41**, 599–604.

Stuart, A. E., Davidson, A. E. and Cumming, R. A. (1967). *J. reticuloendothel. Soc.* **4**, 109–121.

Subrahmanyan, T. P. and Mims, C. A. (1970). *J. reticuloendothel. Soc.* **7**, 32–42.

Suter, E. and Hulliger, L. (1960). *Ann. N.Y. Acad. Sci.* **88**, 1237–1244.

Sutton, J. S. (1967). *Natn. Cancer Inst. Monogr.* **26**, 71–141.

Sutton, J. S. and Weiss, L. (1965). *J. Cell Biol.* **28**, 303–332.

Swartzendruber, D. C. and Congdon, C. C. (1963). *J. Cell Biol.* **19**, 641–646.

Szakal, A. K. and Hanna, M. G. (1968). *Expl. molec. Path.* **8**, 75–89.

Tanaka, H. (1958). *Ann. Rep. Inst. Virus Res. Kyoto Ser. A.* **1**, 87–149.

Tanaka, Y., Epstein, L. N., Brecher, G. and Stohlman, F. (1966). *Blood* **22**, 614–629.

Teoh, T. B. (1961). *J. Path. Bact.* **81**, 33–44.

Thomas, C. E. (1967). *Am. J. Anat.* **120**, 526–552.

Thompson, J. and van Furth, R. (1970). *J. exp. Med.* **131**, 429–442.

Thorbecke, G. J., Old, L. J., Benacerraf, B. and Clarke, D. A. (1963). *J. Histochem. Cytochem.* **8**, 392–399.

Tompkins, E. H. (1946). *Archs Path.* **42**, 299–319.

Tompkins, E. H. (1955). *Ann. N.Y. Acad. Sci.* **59**, 732–745.

Tonna, E. A. (1961). *Anat. Rec.* **137**, 251–270.

Tonna, E. A. (1963). *Nature, Lond.* **200**, 226–227.

Toro, I. (1967). *Meth. Achiev. exp. Path.* **3**, 306–339.

Toro, I. and Rohlich, P. (1962). *Acta Morphol. Acad. Sci. Hung.* **11**, 414–432.

Toro, I., Ruzsa, P. and Rohlich, P. (1962). *Expl. Cell Res.* **26**, 601–603.

Treadwell, P. E. and Santos-Buch, C. A. (1968). *Am. J. Path.* **51**, 483–503.

Unanue, E. R. (1968). *Nature, Lond.* **218**, 36.

Unanue, E. R., Askonas, B. A. and Allison, A. C. (1969). *J. Immunol.* **103**, 71–78.

Unanue, E. R. and Cerottini, J. C. (1970). *J. exp. Med.* **131**, 711–725.

Unanue, E. R., Cerottini, J. C. and Bedford, M. (1969). *Nature, Lond.* **222**, 1193–1195.

Ungar, J. and Wilson, G. R. (1935). *Am. J. Path.* **11**, 681–692.

Vaes, G. (1969). *In* "Lysosomes in Biology and Pathology" (Dingle, J. T. & Fell, H. B., eds), North Holland, Amsterdam.

van Furth, R. (1970). *In* "The Mononuclear Phagocyte." (van Furth, R. ed.). Blackwells, London.

van Furth, R. and Cohn, Z. A. (1968). *J. exp. Med.* **128**, 415–435.

van Furth, R. and Dulk, M. M. C. D-D. (1970). *J. exp. Med.* **132**, 813–828.

van Furth, R., Hirsch, J. G. and Fedorko, M. E. (1970). *J. exp. Med.* **132**, 794–805.

Vaughan, R. B. (1965). *Br. J. exp. Path.* **46**, 71–81.

Vaughan, R. B. and Boyden, S. U. (1964). *Immunology* **7**, 118–126.

Vernon-Roberts, B. (1969a). *Nature, Lond.* **222**, 1286–1288.
Vernon-Roberts, B. (1969b). *Int. Rev. Cytol.* **25**, 131–159.
Virolainen, M. (1968). *J. exp. Med.* **127**, 943–952.
Volkman, A. (1966). *J. exp. Med.* **124**, 241–254.
Volkman, A. and Gowmans, J. L. (1965a). *Br. J. exp. Path.* **46**, 50–61.
Volkman, A. and Gowans, J. L. (1965b). *Br. J. exp. Path.* **46**, 62–70.
Von Kupffer, C. (1876). *Arch. mikrosk. Anat.* **12**, 353–358.

Wachstein, M. (1963). *In* "The Liver", Vol. 2, pp. 137–194. Academic Press, New York and London.
Wanstrup, J. and Christensen, H. E. (1966). *Acta path. microbiol. scand.* **66**, 169–189.
Ward, P. A. (1968). *J. exp. Med.* **128**, 1201–1221.
Watanabe, I., Donahue, S. and Hoggart, N. (1967). *J. Ultrastruct. Res.* **20**, 366–382.
Watanabe, Y. (1965). *Tohoku J. exp. Med.* **89**, 167–176.
Weber, R. (1963). *In* "Lysosomes" (de Reuck, A. V. R. & Cameron, M. P., eds), Churchill, London.
Weiss, L. (1957). *J. biophys. biochem. Cytol.* **3**, 599–609.
Weiss, L. (1959). *J. Anat.* **93**, 465–477.
Weiss, L. (1961). *Bull. Johns Hopk. Hosp.* **108**, 171–199.
Weiss, L. (1962). *Am. J. Anat.* **111**, 131–175.
Weiss, L. (1963a). *Am. J. Anat.* **113**, 51–59.
Weiss, L. (1963b). *Anat. Rec.* **145**, 413–438.
Weiss, L. (1964). *Bull. Johns Hopk. Hosp.* **115**, 99–173.
Weiss, L. (1965). *J. Cell Biol.* **25**, pt. 2, 149–177.
Weiss, L. (1966a). *In* "Histology" (Greep, R. O., ed.), pp. 394–419. McGraw Hill, New York and London.
Weiss, L. (1966b). *J. Morph.* **117**, 467–538.
Weiss, L. and Fawcett, D. W. (1953). *J. Histiochem. Cytochem.* **1**, 47–65.
Wells, A. G. and Carmichael, E. A. (1930). *Brain* **5**, 1–10.
Wennberg, E. and Weiss, L. (1968). *Blood* **31**, 778–790.
White, R. G. (1963). *In* "The Immunologically Competent Cell: Its Nature and Origin" (Wolstenholme, G. E. W. & Knight, J., eds), pp. 6–20, Churchill, London.
Whitelaw, D. M. (1966). *Blood* **28**, 455–464.
Wiener, J. (1967). *In* "The Reticuloendothelial System and Atherosclerosis" (Diluzio, N. R. & Paoletti, R., eds), pp. 85–97. Plenum Press, New York.
Wiener, J. D., Spiro, D. and Russel, P. S. (1963). *Am. J. Path.* **44**, 319–347.
Wiener, J., Spiro, D. and Zunker, H. O. (1965). *Am. J. Path.* **47**, 723–763.
Wiener, J., Cottrell, T. S., Margaretten, W. and Spiro, D. (1967). *Am. J. Path.* **50**, 187–201.
Wilkinson, P. C., Borel, J. F., Stecher-Levin, V. J. and Sorkin, E. (1969). *Nature, Lond.* **222**, 244–247.
Wilkinson, P. J., and Cater, D. B. (1969). *J. Path. Bact.* **97**, 219–230.
Williams, M. A. and Carr, I. (1968). *Expl. Cell Res.* **51**, 196–210.

Williams, W. J., Erasmus, D. A., James, E. M. J. and Davies, T. (1970). *Postgrad. med. J.* **46,** 496–500.
Willoughby, D. A., Coote, E. and Spector, W. G. (1967). *Immunology* **12,** 165–178.
Wisse, E. (1970). *J. Ultrastruct. Res.* **31,** 125–150.
Wisse, E. (1972). *J. Ultrastruct. Res.* **38,** 528–562.
Wisse, E. and Daems, W. Th. (1970). *In* "Mononuclear Phagocytes", pp. 200–209. Blackwell, Oxford.
With, T. K. (1968). "Bile Pigments: Chemical, Biological and Technical Aspects." Academic Press, New York and London.
Wolff, K. (1967). *J. Cell Biol.* **35,** 468–473.
Wolfgram, F. and Rose, A. S. (1957). *J. Neuropath. exp. Neurol.* **16,** 514–531.
Wood, R. L. (1963). *Z. Zellforsch. Mikrosk. Anat.* **58,** 679–692.
Wynn, R. M. (1967). *Am. J. Obstet. Gynec.* **97,** 235–248.
Wyssokowitch, W. (1887). *Z. Hyg. Infekt.-Kr.* **1,** 3.

Yamagishi, M. (1959). *Arch. histol. Jap.* **18,** 223–261.
Yamori, T. and Mori, Y. (1964). *Tohoku J. exp. Med.* **81,** 330–339.
Yamori, T. and Mori, Y. (1967). *Tohoku J. exp. Med.* **91,** 367–374.
Yarborough, O. J., Meyer, O. T., Dannenberg, A. M. and Pearson, B. (1967). *J. reticuloendothel. Soc.* **4,** 390–408.
Young, J. S. (1928). *J. Path. Bact.* **31,** 265–275.

Zamboni, L. and Pease, D. C. (1961). *J. Ultrastruct. Res.* **5,** 65–85.
Zemel, H., Deeken, J., Asel, N. and Packer, J. (1970). *Archs. Path.* **89,** 111–118.
Zucker-Franklin, D., Davidson, M. and Thomas, L. (1966). *J. exp. Med.* **124,** 533–541.
Zwillenberg, I. O. and Zwillenberg, H. I. (1962). *Experientia* **18,** 136–137.

Additional References added in Proof.

Allison, A. C., Davies, P. and de Petris, S. (1971). *Nature New Biol.* **232,** 153–155.
Brederoo, P. and Daems, W.Th. (1972). *Z. Zellforsch. mikrosk. Anat.* **126,** 136–156.
Carr, I. and McGinty, F. (1973). *J. Path.* (in press).
Carr, I. and Underwood, J. C. E. (1973). *Int. Rev. Cytol.* (in press).
Carr, I., Underwood, J. C. E., McGinty, F. and Wood, P. (1973). *J. Path.* (in press).
Chambers, R. C. and Weiser, R. S. (1971). *Cancer Res.* **31,** 2059–2066.
Chambers, R. C. and Weiser, R. S. (1972). *Cancer Res.* **32,** 413–419.
Emeis, J. J. and Wisse, E. (1971). *In* "The Reticuloendothelial System and Immune Phenomena" (N. R. DiLuzio, ed.). Plenum, New York.
Fisher, E. R. and Fisher, B. (1972). *Arch. Path.* **94,** 137–146.
Hard, G. C. and Butler, W. H. (1971). *Cancer Res.* **31,** 337–347.
Lejeune, F. and Evans, R. (1972). *Eur. J. Cancer* **8,** 549–565.

Slatis, P. (1958). *Scand J. clin. Lab. Invest.* **10,** supp. 33, 1–59.

Spritzer, A. A. and Watson, J. A. (1964). *Hlth. Phys.* **10,** 1093–1097

Spritzer, A. A., Watson, J. A., Auld, J. A. and Guetthoff, M. A. (1968). *Archs envir. Hlth* **17,** 726

Underwood, J. C. E. and Carr, I. (1972). *Virchows Archiv. Abt. B. Zellpath.* **12,** 39–50.

Author Index

Numbers in *italics* refer to the pages on which references are listed at the end of each chapter.

Subject Index